THE PERIOD BRAIN

THE
PERIOD BRAIN

The New Science
of Why We PMS and How to Fix It

A MANIFESTO FOR WOMEN

SARAH E. HILL, PhD

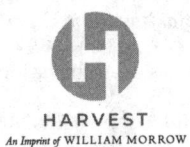

HARVEST
An Imprint of WILLIAM MORROW

Without limiting the exclusive rights of any author, contributor or the publisher of this publication, any unauthorized use of this publication to train generative artificial intelligence (AI) technologies is expressly prohibited. HarperCollins also exercise their rights under Article 4(3) of the Digital Single Market Directive 2019/790 and expressly reserve this publication from the text and data mining exception.

This book contains advice and information relating to health care. It should be used to supplement rather than replace the advice of your doctor or another trained health professional. If you know or suspect you have a health problem, it is recommended that you seek your physician's advice before embarking on any medical program or treatment. All efforts have been made to assure the accuracy of the information contained in this book as of the date of publication. This publisher and the author disclaim liability for any medical outcomes that may occur as a result of applying the methods suggested in this book.

THE PERIOD BRAIN. Copyright © 2025 by Sarah E. Hill. All rights reserved. Printed in the United States of America. No part of this book may be used or reproduced in any manner whatsoever without written permission except in the case of brief quotations embodied in critical articles and reviews. For information, address HarperCollins Publishers, 195 Broadway, New York, NY 10007. In Europe, HarperCollins Publishers, Macken House, 39/40 Mayor Street Upper, Dublin 1, D01 C9W8, Ireland.

HarperCollins books may be purchased for educational, business, or sales promotional use. For information, please email the Special Markets Department at SPsales@harpercollins.com.

hc.com

FIRST EDITION

Designed by Chloe Foster

Illustrations by Katja Cunningham

Library of Congress Cataloging-in-Publication Data has been applied for.

ISBN 978-0-06-338247-3

25 26 27 28 29 LBC 5 4 3 2 1

For you

CONTENTS

Introduction   ix

PART I
The Female Mystery:
Hormones and "Disordered" Women

1. WHY DO WE ALL HAVE PMS?
A neuroendocrinological mystery hidden in plain sight

3

2. UNDERSTANDING YOUR CYCLE
The two halves of your hormonal whole

10

3. HOW IGNORING PROGESTERONE CREATED PMS
Estrogen is about sex and progesterone is about . . . disorder?

24

4. THE DAWN OF BIKINI SCIENCE
Why everything you thought you knew about "normal" is probably male

38

PART II

Reclaiming Female: Rethinking PMS and Embracing Hormonal Change

5. UNDERSTANDING THE LUTEAL PHASE
Progesterone creates unique physical and psychological needs

53

6. IS THERE A METHOD TO YOUR MADNESS?
The upside to feeling down

63

7. SEX AND ATTRACTION ON PROGESTERONE
The great disordering of the female sexual response

85

8. NUTRITION, EXERCISE, SLEEP, AND RECOVERY
Advice for the luteal phase

106

9. FROM PMS TO PRIMARY CARE
Mystery symptoms, mental health, and premenstrual exacerbation of . . . everything

126

10. WHEN A GOOD HORMONE GOES BAD
Answers and support for those with PMDD

146

PART III

The Future Is Female and Hormonal: Welcome to the Revolution

11. RECLAIMING YOUR LUTEAL PHASE
How to promote hormonal balance
177

12. THE FUTURE IS SEX DIFFERENTIATED AND HORMONAL
The end of bikini science
213

Appendix A   231
Appendix B   234
Appendix C   236
Appendix D   238
Acknowledgments   241
Notes   243
Index   273

INTRODUCTION

If you are a woman picking up this book, I'm guessing you have some firsthand experience with feeling terrible premenstrually. Most of us do. The hormonal changes that you experience in the week or two leading up to the start of your period can make you feel overwhelmed and emotional. Gross and unlovable. Hungry and bloated. Irritable and tired. Or maybe you'd describe your premenstrual feelings to me the way they were recently expressed by two women whose responses to my question "How do you feel in the two weeks leading up to the start of your period?" were simply *"Inner scream"* and *"Everyone hates me."*

Ouch.

These women are far from being alone in their struggle to feel good in the last two weeks of their cycle. Most women in the world (including me) have had the experience of feeling like they are riding a premenstrual roller coaster every month that makes us feel less than amazing. Although experiences vary from woman to woman and month to month, most women find themselves feeling some distasteful blend of physical, psychological, and behavioral changes that can include things like feeling irritable, anxious, snacky, tired, bloated, and gross. And, interestingly enough, few of us ever question why. We just assume that this is our fate as women.

So, why do we all feel like sh*t in the weeks leading up to the start of our periods? And is it actually necessary? This is what I have spent the last several years of my life trying to figure out. Because biologically, it doesn't make a whole lot of sense that women should have inherited a tendency to feel bad half the time. And it makes even less sense when you consider that the hormone at the heart of women's terrible experiences each month, progesterone, is actually supposed to make us feel *good*. Despite being deeply entrenched in research on the nuances of all things women and hormones, I had no answers for this. And the more time I spent digging into the literature, the clearer it became that no one else had a really good answer for it either. It was a biological mystery hiding in plain sight. Getting to the bottom of this mystery and telling you about the surprising things I discovered is why I wrote this book. What I learned transformed the way I think about myself and has gotten me off the premenstrual roller coaster. I am hopeful it will have the same effect on you.

First, a bit about me. I am an award-winning research psychologist who studies health and relationships, with a particular focus on women. I have published nearly one hundred scientific research articles on topics in health psychology, evolutionary psychology, and neuroscience. My research is regularly funded by federal grants and discussed in the media, and I am considered a thought leader in the area of women's hormones and psychology. I am passionate about demystifying the results of scientific research and using it to help women understand themselves. As part of these efforts, I authored *This Is Your Brain on Birth Control* (a book about the effects of hormonal birth control on women's brains), I speak and consult on topics related to women's hormonal health, and I serve on the advisory boards for women's health companies like Flo Health and 28 Wellness. I tell you these things to orient you to my background but also to help you understand how elusive the issue of PMS actually is. Because if someone like me doesn't have a clue about why women end up in a socioemotional black hole every month, what hope does it leave for anyone who doesn't have the luxury of being able to sit around and think about hormones all day?

As you will see in the pages to come, everything we experience in the last weeks of the cycle—this thing we call PMS—actually makes biological sense. And it's the sort of biological sense that doesn't require us to feel icky two weeks out of every month. Although the way out of this ickiness is a little more complex than *take two of these and call me in the morning*, it's still very doable. It just requires wrapping our arms around the fact that our female bodies are different from male bodies. And as a part of that differentness, we have to contend with the fact that (a) we have two primary sex hormones instead of one, (b) these hormones cycle, and (c) as our hormones change across the cycle, our bodies' needs change too. This means that the way we have all been taught to think about how our bodies work (as a fixed system instead of a cycling process) is wrong. It also means that the one-size-fits-all information that we have been given about what our bodies need doesn't always fit for us.

Each month, our bodies shift between states dominated by two different and, in many ways, opposing hormones. There is estrogen, the hormone that takes the lead during the first two weeks of the cycle, called the follicular phase. Then there is progesterone, the hormone that takes the lead during the last two weeks of the cycle, called the luteal phase. These hormonal changes matter because they are part of who we are. They *change* us. They create two biologically distinct versions of what the female body is supposed to look like. Estrogen creates a version of ourselves that is optimized for sex and conception. Progesterone creates a version of ourselves that is optimized for implantation and pregnancy. Each of these hormonal states is characterized by distinct patterns of energy expenditure (how many calories we burn), sexual desire, pain perception, threat sensitivity, and more. This means that our bodies' response to everything ranging from the tone in our partner's voice to prescription drugs can—and often does—change over the course of the cycle.

Unfortunately, science has chosen to focus research efforts only on women when we are in the cycle phase dominated by estrogen. This means all of the information we have been given about how to take care of ourselves and what our bodies need was not created with any guidance about what our bodies need or how they behave in the cycle phase dominated by progesterone. And the reason that so many of us feel terrible during this time is because we've been unwittingly fighting against our bodies when they are doing exactly what they are supposed to be doing. It's no wonder we all have PMS.

I wrote this book to change this for you. To help you understand how your body works and what it needs during the half of the cycle that science and medicine typically ignore. To do this, we are going to take a deep dive into the science of progesterone and the luteal phase. We're going to talk about the fascinating complexity of what our bodies are trying to do at this time and how we can support them to feel our best.

Although most of us don't know anything about progesterone, it's an incredible hormone with a fascinating range of effects on our bodies. It's known to affect our daily sleep and calorie needs, our moods, who we're attracted to, the nature of our sexual desire, our ability to read others' emotional states, our ability to put on muscle mass from exercise, our pain perception, our responses to therapy, our responses to prescription drugs, and the severity of our symptoms of just about everything. We will talk about who we are, what our bodies need, and, importantly, how to support our cycles and smooth out the turbulence that can occur in response to our hormonal changes across the cycle. Although this is a cycle phase when women's bodies' needs and vulnerabilities change, there is no reason that most of us should feel as bad as we do.

This book is also going to serve as a rallying cry for all of us to change the way we think about our sex hormones. Many of us have been taught to believe that the most feminist thing we can do when it comes to our sex hormones is pretend they don't matter, but I hope to convince you that it's time to revise this position. Downplaying the impact of our hormones doesn't slow the pace of sexism* or make

---

* Sexist a**sholes will be sexist a**holes regardless of what science has to say. People will always turn a blind eye to the facts when they are trying to stick to an indefensible position. This is why climate change denial is so common despite the fact that there is a huge body of research demonstrating that this is what is on the horizon.

the world a better place for women. Instead, it provides science with an all-too-convenient excuse to continue to mismanage the way we are handled in research and medicine in the name of convenience and saving costs. Rather than studying women as hormonal, the current gold standard in biomedical research is to systematically exclude women from studies when they are in the luteal phase of the cycle to minimize the impact of their hormones on outcomes. And I am guessing you also didn't know that in animal research the females are often ovariectomized so that they don't produce sex hormones at all. Removing sex hormones from what it means to be female totally undermines the spirit behind including female animals in research in the first place. It means women will continue to be in the dark about who they are and what their bodies need when in a high hormonal state, especially in the luteal phase. We'll talk about how science needs to study women *as* women, which means studying us as our hormones cycle.

This book is one part science, one part PMS self-help, and one part exposé on how science has mishandled women. You're going to learn new things about your hormones, about yourself, and about how science works. Learning everything that I have learned in the process of researching and writing this book has changed the way I see myself and has been a total game changer in how I feel. I am confident it will have the same effect on you.

As one final note before we dive in, I want to address the fact that, although much of the research that will be presented in this book focuses on cisgender, heterosexual women, this choice isn't because I believe this is the only—or most important—experience of being a woman. It's because most of the research we have on sex hormones, behavior, and the menstrual cycle overwhelmingly focuses on this population.

It's my hope that this book contributes to a broader conversation about understanding bodies, biology, and lived experiences in all their complexity. The science is a starting point, not the end point. So, while the data I'll present will often focus on the experiences of the cis-het majority, the ultimate goal is to expand what we know and who we listen to, ensuring that all voices are included in shaping the future of this science. You are welcome here, and your curiosity and perspective matter, no matter how closely—or loosely—you fit the mold of the studies I'll be discussing. As I always encourage those who feel like science isn't speaking to their experiences: Be part of the change you'd like to see. Push for better science that is able to tell your story. Better yet, become a scientist. We need your perspective to ensure that science serves all people's needs.

I have spent the last several years of my life uncovering the fascinating science of progesterone and the luteal phase, probing into what it means to be a biological female during a time in the cycle when so many of us feel awful. As you'll see, progesterone—this quiet little hormone that's been sitting at the back of the class and never gets called on—is at the heart of a lot of the things we wrestle with as women. But the problem isn't what progesterone does or who it makes us become. The problem is that we haven't been paying any attention to it. This book is going to be your first step toward changing all of that.

So, let's get started. It's time to discover who we all become in the two weeks of the cycle that the world decided to ignore.

PART I

THE FEMALE MYSTERY

Hormones and "Disordered" Women

CHAPTER 1

WHY DO WE ALL HAVE PMS?

A neuroendocrinological mystery hidden in plain sight

Have you ever thought about how weird it is that most women feel like sh*t in the week or two before their periods start? And how much weirder it is that we all just assume it's inevitable? I literally can't think of anything else in the human experience that is so ubiquitously unpleasant yet assumed to be normal. I mean, childbirth and pain from injury are both universally unpleasant, but they make logical sense. Childbirth hurts because in the evolutionary-size war of babies versus vaginas, babies always win. And pain from injury feels bad to keep us from injuring ourselves further or doing it again. But PMS? Where is the sense in that? If men felt the way we do two weeks out of every month, science and medicine would be working around the clock to direct all available resources toward finding a solution to their suffering. But for us? It's just assumed to be part of the female experience.

So is it? Are women really supposed to be feel some version of awful roughly 50 percent of their adult lives?

Well, if we define normal as something that happens to most people, then PMS *is* normal. Research finds that 75–90 percent of reproductive-age women have it. They report feeling physically and psychologically less well in the week or two leading up to their periods than they do outside that window.

And even though we might think PMS is a privileged-white-lady-with-too-much-time-on-her-hands sort of problem, research finds it's not just white Western women who feel terrible premenstrually. Research finds that women on all six habitable continents around the world show a consistent pattern of feeling worse in the last two weeks of their cycle than they do in the first two.

For example, in one recent study, researchers looked at data from 3.3 million women living in 109 countries around the world to evaluate mood changes across the cycle. Below, you can see the mood map they created based on women's responses. Regions in white show the areas where women reported more happiness and better mood premenstrually. Regions in dark colors show areas where women reported less happiness and worse mood premenstrually. Regions with black dots are areas where there were no mood differences premenstrually. And striped regions are those for which there wasn't enough data.

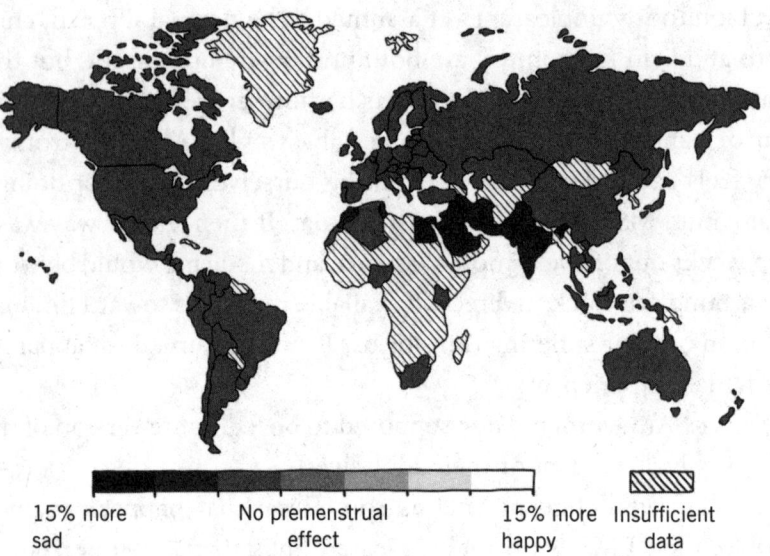

PREMENSTRUAL MOOD EFFECTS

15% more sad — No premenstrual effect — 15% more happy — Insufficient data

Even though you are likely as unsurprised at these results as I was, we should all be appalled by our collective complacency in accepting this depressing mood map as our fate. Because the idea that this is just how things are supposed to be feels defeatist. How is it that we live in a world so rich with possibility that we have self-driving cars and food delivery robots, yet no one has ever bothered to ask whether it is necessary for women to feel bad in the week(s) leading up to the start of their periods?

Why do we feel so universally bad in the week or two before our periods? And is it necessary for us to feel this way?

These are the questions that have been bugging me for years. And not just as a person who has hated feeling like sh*t half the month because I had PMS. They bugged me as a scientist. Because in the world of evolutionary biology, there is nothing about the experience of PMS that makes any sense whatsoever. The idea that reproductive-age women are supposed to go through half of their adult lives feeling awful is evolutionarily bizarre and, frankly, nonsensical. Traits that make people feel awful in their peak reproductive years usually get eliminated from the population because they impinge on our ability to survive and reproduce. This makes them less likely to be inherited than traits that don't cause problems. That is how natural selection works. So, the idea that most of us inherited PMS—in addition to being a total bullsh*t deal for women—is something that the evolutionary biologist in me has never known what to do with.

One possibility I considered is that PMS might be an inevitable side effect of having cycles. And that the reason it persists is because it isn't costly enough for natural selection to remove from the population. Sort of like a belly button—it serves no purpose but also causes no real harm. Maybe PMS is just a meaningless by-product of the hormonal changes we experience each month that hasn't caused enough problems for evolution to decouple the terrible feelings we have premenstrually from the hormonal changes it's associated with.*

---

* Note that for the process of evolution by selection to be able to decouple the tendency to feel terrible from the hormonal changes that happen at the end of the cycle would require there to be sufficient variability in how women feel in response to these hormonal changes. If there were no women who felt just fine in response

As appealing as this argument sounded at first, the more time I spent with it, the clearer it became that it wasn't very plausible. While PMS might not pose the same type of survival threat as something like cancer or cardiovascular disease, it's hardly uncostly. PMS and period-related symptoms are responsible for an average of 8.9 days of lost work productivity per woman per year. Women who suffer from PMS are more likely to experience low self-esteem and relationship difficulties than nonsufferers. All in, researchers estimate that the impact of PMS on women's quality of life and economic functioning is comparable to major depressive disorder. And for women with PMDD (premenstrual dysphoric disorder), these impacts can even cost them their lives. The risk of suicidality in these women is seven times higher than what it is for nonsufferers.

So, PMS isn't just costly. It's super costly. And even though our ancestors cycled a lot less frequently than we do now (they were too busy being pregnant and lactating to have as many cycles as we do), there is simply no way that the overwhelming majority of contemporary women would have inherited this costly predisposition if it wasn't providing us with some sort of benefit that could outweigh these enormous costs.

Another explanation I considered is the possibility that PMS isn't something that our female ancestors had to deal with at all. Maybe all the terrible feelings we saw splayed across the premenstrual mood map are the result of all the environmental changes we've made in the last hundred years that mess with our hormones. The quality of the human diet has gone down and exposure to toxic chemicals has gone up since the time of our ancestors. So, if these changes correspond to changing rates of PMS, it could be that it is a disease of civilization, like type 2 diabetes and heart disease.

---

to end-of-cycle hormonal changes, evolution could never select against the tendency to feel terrible. However, such variability does exist. There are some women who experience no premenstrual yuckiness, some who experience only marginal levels, and some who experience hugely terrible levels. There is enough variability for selection to work on this trait.

Although there was a lot to like about this explanation, it also failed to connect all the dots. While it is true that the modern environment and all its exposures don't do us any favors premenstrually (more on this in chapter 11), this isn't the only reason we feel bad. PMS isn't just something that happens to women fortunate enough to live in countries with terrible diets and an overreliance on plastics. It happens to all of us. And research on nonhuman animals finds evidence of PMS-like symptoms in species ranging from rats to baboons. For example, female yellow baboons (*Papio cynocephalus*) are less social and more combative with peers premenstrually than at other times in the cycle. Others find that creating a hormonal state that mimics PMS causes rats and mice to exhibit increases in anxiety-like behavior. Premenstrual changes in anxiety and aggression are also observed in vervet monkeys and even dairy cows, suggesting that PMS may have less to do with where we live and what we're exposed to than it does to the fact that we're female and experience hormonal changes each month.

This brings us back to square one. Why do females great and small routinely feel bad in the weeks leading up to their periods? And why, despite the growing public awareness of menstrual cycles and hormonal changes, hasn't anyone spent time trying to figure out what our bodies need at this time to help us feel better? There are many books and other resources talking about the fertile window and how wonderful and magical estrogen makes us feel. And while this is great and all, most of us don't need a survival guide to help navigate the experience of feeling awesome. We need one that tells us what to do when we're feeling bad. And currently there is almost no conversation around what most of us experience in the second half of the cycle or the sex hormone progesterone, which is at the heart of everything we feel at this time.

The more I began to dig into these issues to try to unwind the neuroendocrinological and evolutionary principles behind them, the clearer it became that PMS is an inevitable consequence of experiencing hormonal changes in a world that was not created with female bodies in mind. It's biology and sexism in equal measure. PMS is one part functional biological changes that happen on purpose and make us feel different in the last two weeks of the cycle than we do in the first. And it's one part dysfunctional changes resulting from the fact that most of us are unknowingly eating, sleeping, exercising, and socializing according to advice that works in the first half of our cycle, but not the second. No one has taught us that our bodies' needs change throughout the month. And no one has taught us that when we try to care for ourselves following guidance that only works for our bodies half the time, it's going to make us feel awful.

Here are five things about PMS that have become crystal clear to me over the last several years:

- **The luteal phase has a purpose.** Many of the physical, psychological, and behavioral changes that occur in the last two weeks of our cycles reflect changes that happen *on purpose*. And we have inherited them because they provided important benefits to our female ancestors. Seriously. There is a method to at least some of the madness.
- **Progesterone is the hormone at the heart of these feelings.** These on-purpose changes are prompted by the rise and fall of the sex hormone progesterone, which floods our brains and bodies during the second two weeks of our cycle before our periods arrive.
- **Women aren't disordered; we have just been ignored by science.** Ignoring our cyclicity has *created* disorder. PMS is the tip of a much larger iceberg encompassing ways that women have suffered because our changing needs across the cycle—specifically those occurring in the two weeks leading up to our periods—have been ignored by science and medicine.
- **Our environment plays a role.** Environmental changes that we have made in the last hundred years or so have both decreased our exposure to progesterone and made us more sensitive to hormonal changes, both of which can contribute to physical and psychological turbulence during this time.

- **You can feel better:** Giving women the information they need to support their bodies during the luteal phase and other periods of hormonal transition can ease distress and leave them feeling a lot better.

This is what we are going to be spending our time together talking about in the pages of this book. And it's about time. Half the world's population has no business feeling terrible half the time. When you change the way you think about your cycle and begin to embrace each of the distinct halves to the female hormonal whole, it can put you on a path to feeling so much better.

Although most of us know about our periods, our hormonal changes don't just affect us from the waist down. They affect *everything*. This includes our moods, our energy levels, our calorie needs, our sexual interest and responsiveness, our taste in partners, and how our bodies respond to physical pain, exercise, immunological threats, and even psychotherapy. They. Affect. Everything. And this includes our very sense of who we are. When our hormones go through changes, it changes the way we experience the world.

Let's dive into the science of our cycles and sex hormones. As you'll see, although our hormones change across the cycle, these changes don't need to be the source of our suffering. And if we nurture our cycles instead of trying to fight them, ignore them, or medicate them out of existence, most of us can feel a whole lot better than we do right now.

CHAPTER 2

UNDERSTANDING YOUR CYCLE

The two halves of your hormonal whole

If you're anything like me, I'm guessing that you didn't get much of a hormonal education growing up. I mean, I'm sure we all saw the same awful puberty video in fifth grade. And maybe your mom told you that your hormones can make you feel more emotional during your period. But for most women I know (including me), the extent to which we were taught about our hormones and the important role they play in our mental and physical health never went much further than that.

So, before we can get to the bottom of PMS, the first thing we have to do is get acquainted with how our hormones work.*

Hormones are chemical messengers in your body whose job it is to get all your cells marching in the same direction toward goals set by the brain. In short, when the brain says "[insert name of some goal here]," your hormones are part of the marching orders that are

---

* If you're already well versed in the ins and outs of the endocrine system (or have read my first book), you can probably skip to the end of this chapter. What we are going to go over here is pretty entry-level, Hormones 101 type of stuff. For those of you who haven't received any sort of hormonal self-education, though, these pieces will be helpful to you as we continue to march our way through the remaining chapters of this book.

sent throughout the body to help accomplish that goal. For example, if you haven't eaten in a while, your brain will call for the release of hunger hormones to get your body's wheels in motion for finding and consuming food. Or if we get a hug from a friend, our brain will release hormones like oxytocin and dopamine, which help flag our friend as being one of our people and help reinforce that they are someone who should be treated with more love, generosity, and forgiveness than we offer most others in our life.

As master coordinators of all our body's parts, hormones are a part of the physiological software programs that create the experience of being you. Whether it's growth and development, eating, drinking, stressing, having sex, maintaining a pregnancy, or bonding with our loved ones, hormones get all your bits and pieces working together to do whatever it is that the brain has in mind.

The communication between the brain and the parts of the body that create and release hormones goes on through a three-part communication pathway that looks a little like this:

Hypothalamus (in your brain) → Pituitary → Endocrine Organ

It starts with the hypothalamus, which is a part of your brain. One of its big jobs is to release special hormones to the pituitary gland, which is a little pea-shaped organ that's right beneath your brain, near the brain stem. These releasing hormones tell the pituitary to stimulate whichever endocrine organ produces the hormone the brain would like released. The pituitary then communicates directly to whichever endocrine organ is being called to duty, ultimately leading to hormone release.

When hormones are released, they go into the bloodstream and go everywhere that blood travels, from head to toe. *Everywhere.*[*] This sort

---

[*] This is why, contrary to what some doctors tell their female patients, the hormonal IUD—which many women use for birth control—does not act locally. You cannot have a locally acting hormone because hormones go everywhere blood goes, which means that the hormones go—you guessed it—everywhere.

of diffuse release is what allows hormonal messages to reach multiple cells, tissues, and organs quickly, efficiently, and all at once. Once in the bloodstream, hormones get picked up by all cells in the body that have receptors for them. This will then cause the cell to change what it is doing based on the messaging the hormone provides.

For example, if a cell is being stimulated by sex hormones, it will do whatever it is supposed to do to help the body prepare for sex and reproduction. If it is stimulated by stress hormones, it will do whatever it is supposed to do to help the body prepare for stress. And if it receives both types of hormones at the same time? Well, it will do whatever it is supposed to do to help the body prepare for stressful sex (or sexy stress . . . whatever that might look like). As master coordinators of physiological processes and behavior, hormones change the activities of lots of different systems within the body at once. Whether you're eating, drinking, fighting, fleeing, stressing, sleeping, sexing, or doing whatever else it is your body might be up to at any given moment, your hormones are part of your body's invisible machinery that makes all this possible. They are part of what makes you *you*. We are our brains. We are our neurotransmitters. And we are our hormones.

The Thing About Sex Hormones

Although we have a lot of important hormones that do a lot of important things in our bodies (I'm looking at you, cortisol and thyroxine), there's a strong case to be made that none of them are quite as important or impactful as our sex hormones. This is because—as a species that's inherited every single trait that we have from sexual reproduction—our brains and bodies are literally wired for sex and pregnancy. And this is true even for those of us who don't want sex or babies. Every trait you have is something you inherited because it was possessed by a female ancestor who (a) had sex and (b) had babies. If even one of your direct ancestors failed to do either of these things, you wouldn't be here. Ancient humans who had sex and babies passed their traits down to descendants. And ancient humans who failed to do these things didn't pass their traits down to anyone.

This process of inheriting traits that promote sex and reproduction (and not inheriting traits that are antagonistic to either pursuit) is called natural selection. And when this process of differential trait inheritance causes changes in gene frequencies over time, it is called evolution. It's important to understand how this process works because it can help us understand why our sex hormones are so important when it comes to calling the shots within our bodies. Without our sex hormones, there'd be no reproduction. And without reproduction, we'd fail to persist as a species. Although most of us think of sex as being nothing more than a pleasurable pastime to be shared with the person (or people) we love (or lust after), it's the engine that has powered our continuity as a species for hundreds of thousands of years. This makes the hormones that coordinate these activities some of the most powerful and influential pieces of molecular machinery our bodies have.

Now, as you might expect from their name, the job of sex hormones is to get all the parts of our body working together to help coordinate sex (and reproduction). And this is true for all of us. But what sex and reproduction actually end up looking like and demand of the body is something that differs in pretty dramatic ways depending on whether you are male or female. Male bodies do one thing; female bodies do another. Although biological sex can seem trivial and unnecessary in an age during which there is growing awareness of gender fluidity, it is at the heart of understanding why women are so hormonally different from men.

Let's start by talking about what biological males must do to reproduce.* And this won't take us very long because the only thing that

---

* From here on out, I am going to drop the "biological" before I talk about biological males and biological females, calling them male and females instead. This is being done in the service of speech economy and does not imply that I assume that all biological females will be female gendered or that biological sex is somehow more important than gender. Neither of these things are true. We are just going to

men need to do to reproduce is have sex.* I mean, of course they have to find a partner first. Then they have to do all the things necessary to get their partner interested in sex. But that's pretty much the extent of what's required of men to get their genes into the next generation. It's one job with three steps: Find a partner, mutually conclude that sex is a fine idea, and then do the deed.

Now, because men only need to jump through one set of hoops to get their genes into the next generation, they only need one primary sex hormone. This sex hormone is called testosterone. And as the hormone charged with coordinating the one job that men's brains and bodies need to do to get their genes into the next generation (sex, sex, and more sex), testosterone is known as a potent motivator of sex (duh), as well as all its various antecedents.

Research finds, for example, that men's testosterone levels are related to just about everything having to do with sex and attraction, including sexual desire, sexual function, their desired number of lifetime sexual partners, their interest in—and success with—attracting serious dating partners, and their interest in—and success with—attracting extra-pair or casual sexual partners. We see these patterns when looking at differences in testosterone levels among men. We see these patterns when looking at changes in testosterone levels occurring within men (for example, in response to changes in the time of day). And we see these patterns in response to testosterone being administered or blocked for clinical or experimental purposes. For example, clinicians regularly report that male-gendered biological females experience strong increases in sexual desire soon after beginning testosterone therapy to affirm their male gender identity. The opposite is found in their female-gendered biological male counterparts taking testosterone-blocking drugs (in combination with es-

---

be talking about biological differences that owe themselves to the sex-differentiated nature of reproduction, which means talking about biological sex.

* Parenting/fathering is a different story. Human men are actually one of the standouts in the animal kingdom in terms of just how much they typically invest in the care and rearing of children.

trogen) to help affirm their female identity. Research conducted on nonhuman animals—such as on songbirds and rats—finds that you can turn sexual behavior on and off like a light switch simply by administering and blocking testosterone.

So, men's primary sex hormone, testosterone, motivates all things sex, including sex (intercourse and all things intercourse-adjacent), as well as behaviors like competing for status, power, and other resources that will make them more competitive in the mating market. For example, testosterone levels predict men's willingness to take risks (whether physical, financial, or business related), how fiercely they compete to win, their preference for wealth-signaling luxury products, and the magnitude of their displays of generosity (particularly toward partners). So, testosterone is all about sex and attraction, which is the one set of activities men's bodies are responsible for to get their genes into the next generation.

Things aren't quite as simple for those of us who are female. Instead of having one job our bodies need to do to get our genes into the next generation, we have two. Like men, our brains and bodies have to invest effort in sex and attraction. So, we need a hormone to help coordinate all of that. But we also have to invest in embryo implantation and pregnancy. Which means we need a hormone to coordinate all of that too. Two jobs. Two hormones.

For women, the sex hormone that's in charge of coordinating all the activities related to sex and attraction is estrogen.* Estrogen, in addition to being the hormone charged with coordinating the development and maintenance of our secondary sexual characteristics (things like breasts, hips, and pubic hair), is also the driver of how sexy we feel, how sexy we appear to others, and our motivation for sex. Estrogen is highest in the cycle during times in which sex can lead

---

* Although testosterone also plays a role in women's sexual desire and functioning (like in men, it promotes sexual desire, sexual function, and the desire to win at competitions), its role is more secondary. Women's testosterone is about twenty times lower than men's. The big driver of all things female sex, sexiness, and attraction is estrogen.

to pregnancy. And, as a result of this, it tells the body to pull out all the physical and psychological stops on all things sex and attraction. We'll talk more about what these things look like in chapter 3.

The second thing that female bodies have to do to reproduce is to actually grow a new human. This means pregnancy, which requires transforming the body into a version of itself that is able to support two living beings instead of one. The sex hormone in charge of this transformation is called progesterone. Progesterone is in charge of thickening the endometrial lining, tamping down the immune system so it doesn't attack any implanting embryos, and prompting other physical and psychological changes that help prepare for the possibility of having to support new life.

Because women's bodies have two jobs to do in reproduction—sex and pregnancy—our sex hormones cycle. They transition our bodies between two distinct physical and psychological states, each of which is optimized to do one of the two jobs required for reproduction.

So, what does this look like?

The estrogenic sex and attraction phase of the cycle is called the follicular phase. It starts on Day 1 of your cycle (which is the day your period starts) and it continues until an egg is released at ovulation (something that usually happens around Day 14-ish). During the first days of the follicular phase, when you're bleeding, hormone levels are super low. Even though women are often given a hard time about being hormonal when they have their periods, this is actually the time in the cycle when our sex hormones are at their lowest (take that, sexist a**holes). These low hormone levels are picked up by the brain (in the hypothalamus), which lets it know that an embryo has not implanted and that it's time to start stimulating egg follicles to prepare for a new round of ovulation. The brain tells the pituitary to stimulate the ovaries to begin maturing egg follicles, which it does through the release of follicle-stimulating hormone (FSH) and luteinizing hormone (LH). The release of these pituitary hormones prompts several egg follicles to begin maturing within one of the ovaries, which causes the release of our first primary sex hormone, estrogen.

Soon after the follicles begin to mature, a dominant follicle will emerge. This role is assumed by the egg follicle that shows the most promise early in development. It will continue to grow and mature while the others retreat and get reabsorbed into the body. As this happens, estrogen levels continue to increase, rising sharply, particularly in the five or so days preceding ovulation. This period of time is known as the fertile window, so named because it is a time when sex can lead to conception (sex can lead to conception roughly five days prior to ovulation and up to twenty-four hours after). Estrogen generally reaches its peak around Day 14 of the cycle, prompting a hormonal cascade that tells the egg to emerge from the follicle and begin its magical journey down the fallopian tube. This is ovulation. And with its occurrence begins the end of the follicular phase of the cycle.

The second half of the cycle—the one responsible for implantation and pregnancy—is known as the luteal phase. It is characterized by release of our second primary sex hormone, progesterone, which gets released after ovulation and remains elevated until the start of your next period.

The luteal phase begins after ovulation occurs. Progesterone gets released from a temporary endocrine structure called the corpus luteum, which forms inside the egg follicle that became vacated at

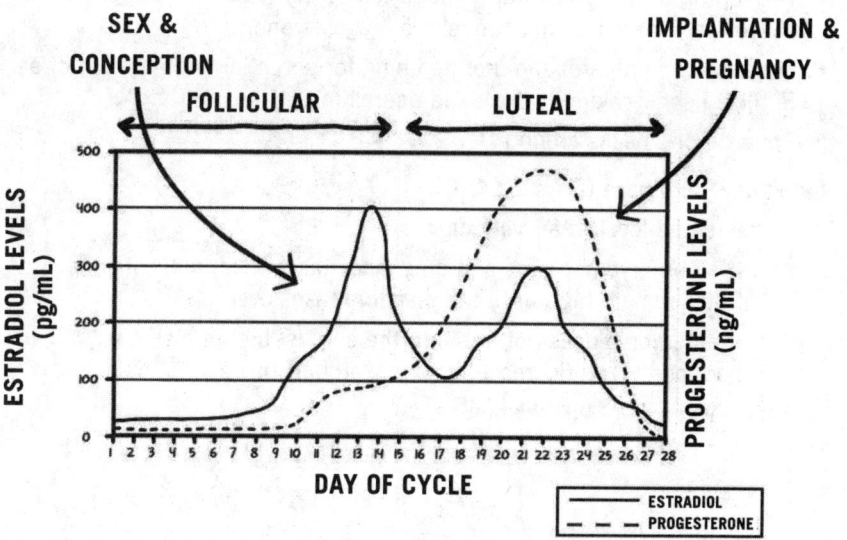

KEY MOMENTS IN YOUR CYCLE: A CHEAT SHEET

FOLLICULAR PHASE

Early follicular phase (Days 1–5-ish when you have your period):
- The day you get your period is Day 1 of your cycle. It is initiated by a big hormone crash at the end of the luteal phase.
- Your sex hormones are at their lowest point in the cycle. This alerts the brain that you are not pregnant, prompting the hormonal cascade that stimulates egg follicles.

Mid-follicular phase (Days 5–9-ish):
- Several egg follicles begin to develop, causing the release of estrogen. The uterine lining thickens.
- One dominant follicle emerges. This is the egg that will ultimately be released. It continues to develop while the others retreat. Estrogen increases steadily.

Fertile window and ovulation (Days 9-ish–14-ish):
- Estrogen is rising, peaking near Day 14 and prompting ovulation.
- Sex can lead to conception during the fertile window, the five-ish days prior to ovulation and up to twenty-four hours after the egg is released.

LUTEAL PHASE

Early and mid-luteal subphase (Days 15–21):
- The ruptured egg follicle turns into a temporary endocrine structure called the corpus luteum. It releases progesterone.
- Progesterone prepares the uterine lining for potential implantation of a fertilized egg, making it thick and nourishing.
- Progesterone peaks around Day 22.

Late luteal subphase (Days 22–28):
- Progesterone levels start very high.
    1. If an embryo implants and pregnancy takes hold, progesterone levels remain high until the placenta takes over.
    2. If an embryo does not implant, the corpus luteum dissolves and hormone levels decrease, crashing around Day 28.
- This is when PMS hits women hard.

ovulation. Progesterone levels rise steadily during the first seven or so days of the luteal phase, usually peaking near Day 22. This peak serves as something of a hormonal punctuation mark on what we call the implantation window, which is the four or five days each month in which the endometrium is open to the possibility of embryo implantation. This generally happens during Day 19–22-ish of a 28-day cycle.

After progesterone's mid-luteal phase peak, levels either (a) remain high and increase because a fertilized egg has implanted and pregnancy has begun or (b) begin to decrease as the corpus luteum starts to disintegrate, leading to a hormone crash that occurs around Day 28, ushering in your period and the start of a new cycle. The luteal phase of the cycle is when women get PMS, which can hit particularly hard during times when progesterone levels are changing most rapidly.

We cycle between those two sex hormones roughly every twenty-eight-ish days, and we do this because our bodies have two jobs to do for reproduction to occur. Two jobs → two hormones → two halves to our hormonal whole.

For Those of You with Irregular Cycles

Although most of us cycle between our two primary sex hormones roughly every twenty-eight days, not everyone has predictable cycles. This is particularly true for women in a hormonal transition space like perimenopause (a precursor to menopause, when our cycles tend to get erratic) or who have issues like polycystic ovarian syndrome (PCOS). Many women experience irregular cycles at some point in their lives, which can make it hard to identify what's going on with themselves hormonally.

If this describes you, my first suggestion is that you try to get it back on track. There are a number of wonderful books out there by people like Lara Briden (*Period Repair Manual*), Nicole Jardim (*Fix Your*

Period), and others who offer help to women with disobedient cycles. I will also talk about ways to support regular ovulation and hormonal health in chapter 11, making this another place to start. Although this recommendation won't do much to help those in the perimenopausal space, everyone can benefit from taking steps to support the cycle.

The second suggestion I have is one that works for all women. And that is to learn how to identify ovulation (which I go over in detail in chapter 11). This will help you identify (a) if and when you're experiencing anovulatory cycles and (b) when you are shifting from the follicular phase to the luteal. Although those of you in perimenopause might roll your eyes at the idea of learning to track your fertility when it is clearly trying to exit stage left, I can honestly say that this skill is far more valuable to me at age forty-six than it was at age thirty-two. Knowing the frequency with which I am ovulating has helped me keep closer tabs on where I am in my transition out of fertility and better predict my periods.

Regardless of why your cycle is irregular, learning to recognize when you are ovulating will allow you to keep track of what's going on hormonally. Once you get your period up until you ovulate, you are in the follicular phase, and your dominant sex hormone is estrogen. And after you ovulate up until you get your next period, you are in the luteal phase and your dominant sex hormone is progesterone.

Everything in Nature Is Natural, Including You

I want to close this chapter by addressing any residual discomfort you might have in response to all the emphasis on (heterosexual) sex and babies when talking about the function of our cycles and our hormones. None of us like to feel that all our interesting complexity is being reduced to our ability to procreate. This is especially true if we are someone whose gender identity, sexual orientation, or lack of motherhood aspirations differ from that of our direct ancestors. And it can feel downright cruel if we are one of the growing numbers of women who had motherhood aspirations that didn't pan out the way we wanted them to. Having definitions of womanhood so tightly intertwined with motherhood can have the unintentional effect of making some among us feel like there is not a place for them in this discussion about our sex hormones and cycles.

I want to take a minute to walk through these issues and for me to assure you that there is a spot for you at this table. We are not on a slow march into a Fox News special where I tell you that women's highest calling is to make and care for babies, and that any deviation from that calling is "unnatural." You don't need to live like your ancestors or share their procreational ambitions and focus to be explainable by biology. Instead, by understanding the things they did that ultimately led to the creation of you, the predilections of our ancestors can help you to understand some of the things about yourself that simply don't make sense otherwise.

Our sex hormones differ from men's because our bodies each play different roles in reproduction. And while it's true that natural selection did its thing by passing down traits that ultimately resulted in sex and babies, this doesn't mean that having sex and babies is what "science" says women should be doing. It also doesn't mean that being a mother is somehow more "natural" than any other choice that a woman might make that deviates from this narrow, limiting path. It just means that many of the female-specific traits we have can be understood because of the role they played in gene transmission.

Regardless of what anyone might try to tell you, there is nothing (*nothing!*) about any choice you might make—no matter how far afield from the heterosexual, barefoot, pregnant path that our ancestors had no choice but to tread—that is unnatural or flies in the face of science. Everything in nature is natural.* And that includes

---

* Yes. Seriously. I would argue that even things like Yellow dye #5 and Red dye #40—while not being things that our ancestors were exposed to—are nonetheless natural because they were ideas borne of the human nervous system. They are products of the brain. So, while inventions like food dye are not natural *foods*

you, your brain, and all the decisions your brain makes. This is true whether the decisions you make are the sort that would have led our ancestors to pass on genes or not. You are nature. You are natural. And there aren't any decisions that you could possibly make that would invalidate that.

And if that isn't enough to convince you that evolutionary theory does not prescribe motherhood to women, let me point out that a deep, burning desire to have children isn't likely something that was actively selected for in women anyway. The reason for this is because for most of human history women didn't have a choice about motherhood. There was no birth control. Motherhood was something that was thrust upon sexually active women whether they wanted to have children or not. This is undoubtedly why so many of us are more ambivalent about motherhood than we are about sex. Having children was the default position for women who were regularly having sex, no desire for motherhood required.*

So, looking at our hormones and cycles through an evolutionary lens is not something that is prescriptive or limiting to women. If it were, there's no way I would have spent my career using these principles as my theoretical tool of choice in trying to understand women and myself. Although my life has been benchmarked by heterosexual sex, pregnancy, and babies (an evolutionary triple play), I've also restricted my fertility with birth control, had a busy career outside the home, and done a whole bunch of other stuff that my ancestors probably wouldn't approve of or couldn't have done themselves. I use these tools of science to understand women because there is simply no other theory out there that is better equipped to help us under-

---

(meaning that our ancestors were never exposed to them, making them outside the scope of foods our bodies are optimized to consume), they are nonetheless natural in the sense that they are products of our big, beautiful, biological brains.

* Interestingly, now that we have access to contraception, this will put selection pressure on the desire for motherhood. Over the next million years, we will likely see an increase in the frequency of women who actively want children because genes related to wanting to be child-free will decrease in frequency.

stand women and their hormones, and why, as our sex hormones change, we change. It's only when we begin to understand the function of the head-to-toe changes our bodies undergo across the cycle that we can begin to understand what our bodies need in the luteal phase and find answers to PMS.

CHAPTER 3

HOW IGNORING PROGESTERONE CREATED PMS

Estrogen is about sex and progesterone is about . . . disorder?

Given what you now know about hormones, it probably won't come as a huge surprise that our brains and bodies can behave pretty differently depending on whether our body is gearing up for sex and conception (estrogen) or implantation and pregnancy (progesterone). When estrogen is the sex hormone calling the shots in the body (the follicular phase), it causes physical and psychological changes that increase both our ability to discriminate between prospective mates and our desire for sex. And when progesterone is the sex hormone calling the shots (the luteal phase), it prompts physical and psychological changes that get our bodies geared up for pregnancy.

This general idea that our sex hormones should prompt coordinated action in the body to help facilitate sex and pregnancy has been really well supported when it comes to the follicular phase and estrogen. Mountains of research studies have been published on species ranging from horses to human beings showing that estrogen is all about sex.

For example, in one study, researchers had 1,066 naturally cycling* women keep daily diaries of their cycle phase and desire for sex for a period of two years. They gathered data on more than twenty thousand different cycles to see whether a relationship exists between estrogen levels across the cycle and women's sexual desire. Their results revealed a striking peak in desire at times in the cycle when estrogen is high and conception possible. And once ovulation had occurred and sex was no longer conceptive (in the luteal phase), they found that women's sexual desire took a nosedive into its cycle-based low.

This general pattern has since been replicated dozens of times in several different studies, including one by my research team in partnership with the scientist researchers at Natural Cycles. In this study, we analyzed user data from more than one thousand (consenting) users of the Natural Cycles fertility tracking app. These users collectively tracked more than five thousand cycles, which we then analyzed for cycle-based changes in both sexual desire and sexual behavior. We found there was a marked increase in women's sexual desire (how much sex they wanted) and sexual behavior (how much sex they were having) at times in the cycle when estrogen is highest and conception is possible. Interestingly, we found these patterns even among those women who were using the app to actively try to *avoid* pregnancy.†

---

* You are going to hear me use the phrase "natural cycling" a lot. Saying a woman is naturally cycling is just shorthand for me saying that she is (a) premenopausal and (b) not on hormonal birth control. Hormonal birth control prevents ovulation, meaning that these women don't have cycles. And, of course, menopausal women don't have cycles either. So a naturally cycling woman is simply a woman who has ovulatory cycles.

† Interestingly, this isn't all that unusual. Our unconscious mind can sometimes play dirty tricks on us and try to convince us to do things that will get us pregnant, even when our conscious mind wants absolutely nothing to do with having a baby. For example, I have had women tell me that they will have thoughts pop into their heads at high fertility, like "Skip the condom! You won't get pregnant anyway!" or "Don't worry about birth control. Having a baby would be EXCITING!" And then after the moment has passed and sex is done, they're shocked by their own stream of consciousness. And they swear that this only happens to them when they're in

Women desire more sex and have more sex at times in the cycle when estrogen is high because this is what their brains want them to do, pregnancy avoidance goals be damned.

Women's sexual motivation and desire increase in the days leading up to ovulation because of rising estrogen levels. Because of this, heterosexual women have more sex near ovulation. Lesbian women have more sex near ovulation. And for those looking for a no-hassle orgasm, masturbation levels increase near ovulation. Sex is something that is on people's minds (and in people's beds) during the fertile window, and estrogen is the driver.

Women's bodies experience changes from head to toe that are all geared toward increasing the probability of conception near ovulation. This is why the estrogenic phase of the cycle is typically a fun, flirty, sexy time for most women. Everything about us changes in ways that promote sex and attraction during the fertile window. This includes the texture of our cervical mucus as well as the scent of our skin, our brain's responses to pleasure, and the way we dress, move, and interact with potential mates.

In one study, for example, researchers had women come into the research lab twice across the course of their cycle: once in the fertile window when estrogen was rising and conception was possible, and once in the luteal phase, when progesterone was rising and sex was no longer conceptive. At each session, women were asked to imagine they were going to a social gathering at a friend's apartment that would be attended by a lot of single, attractive women and men. Women were asked to imagine what they would wear to the event and then asked to draw their outfit of choice on a paper doll using colored pencils provided by the researchers. Afterward, the research team measured the square millimeters of skin that were exposed on the dolls and had an outside group of evaluators rate how sexy the outfits were.

---

the fertile window. Although this is not something that has been tested and verified in research, it is consistent with other work that finds evidence of sex-facilitating self-deception when women are at high fertility across the cycle.

Below, you can see one pair of drawings made by one of the women who participated in the study. The outfit to the left is what she drew when she was in the luteal phase. The outfit to the right was drawn by the same woman near ovulation when conception was possible. And this woman was far from unique in her outfit choices. The study found that the outfits drawn by women near ovulation were significantly sexier and more revealing than the ones drawn by women during the luteal phase.

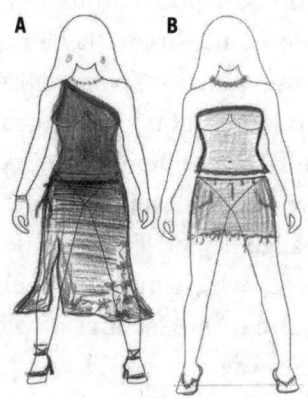

But there's more.

In addition to drawing sexier and more revealing outfits on paper dolls at high fertility compared to low, the women actually *wore* sexier and more revealing outfits to the lab for their high-fertility session. The researchers took pictures of what the women had on when they came to the lab for each of their sessions. And just like they did with the drawings, they had their outfits measured and rated for skin exposure and sexiness. Consistent with what they found when they analyzed the clothing the women drew on their paper dolls, the women actually wore sexier and more revealing clothes at their high-fertility sessions than they did at low.

Estrogen causes the brain and body to become more easily excited, pleasure-primed, sexually engaged versions of themselves. For example, estrogen turns the volume up and down on reward sensitivity in ways that make sex seem more pleasurable and make food seem less so. It increases women's attentional attunement to all things male, increasing women's preference for masculinized faces, voices, and behavioral displays. It also makes women look, feel, and smell like the sexiest versions of themselves to men, making it a hormone that is about both attraction and attracting.

When you look at all the changes that go on in the brain in response to rising levels of estrogen, it's clear to see why patterns like this emerge. Estrogen acts like Miracle-Gro in the nervous system, causing the birth of new dendritic spines on neurons in important areas like the hippocampus, hypothalamus, amygdala, and the prefrontal cortex. These areas of the brain play an important role in things like memory, emotion regulation, personality, and minor details like directing our conscious thoughts. These changes make our brain a more excitable, rapidly responding, memory-forming version of itself than it is when estrogen levels are low. Estrogen also increases the synthesis and availability of feel-good neurotransmitters like serotonin and dopamine, which make us feel good about ourselves, keep anxiety at bay, and create feelings of pleasure, satisfaction, and desire . . . exactly the way we would want a brain to feel at times when sex can lead to conception. We feel on top of our game, full of energy, sexy, and alive because evolution by selection would have it no other way.

When we look at the research on everything that estrogen does to our brains and bodies during this time, it fits really nicely into a narrative about estrogen nudging our brain and body into a state that is optimized for partner choice, sex, and conception. And this makes a lot of evolutionary sense. It doesn't take a huge stretch of the imagination to understand why contemporary women might have inherited a tendency to be primed for sex and pleasure at times in the cycle when sex can lead to pregnancy. Wanting and enjoying sex at times when it can lead to gene transmission is an insanely inheritable trait for anyone to have. And when you look at the research on all of the wonderful things that estrogen does to women's brains and bodies, much of it maps neatly onto the predictions that scientists have made about estrogen's role as being a great facilitator of female sexual behavior.

Progesterone, on the other hand, is a little bit more challenging to understand . . . because there is very little about this hormone or this cycle phase that fits neatly into a box of any kind. Even though this is the sex hormone behind conception and pregnancy, understanding its effects in the brain in relation to these tasks isn't quite as straightforward as it is with estrogen. This is because many of the things that women experience in the luteal phase in response to progesterone—unlike the things they experience in the follicular phase in response to estrogen—don't seem to make a lot of sense in terms of the function they are supposed to be serving. Rather than coordinating a suite of physical, psychological, and behavioral changes that make sense in the context of pregnancy preparation, most of the changes women experience in the context of progesterone just look like . . . PMS. Progesterone seems to be about little more than making us all feel terrible . . . which doesn't really make any sense at all.

To illustrate this point, my research team and I recently asked a sample of 150 naturally cycling women to spend a minute thinking about how they feel the two weeks before their periods start. Then we had them list the things that popped into their heads when they thought about this time. My team then took all the women's responses and turned them into a word cloud, which you can see below. The words that came up most frequently are those that are the largest in the cloud. Smaller words are those that came up less frequently. And words that are absent (e.g., fabulous, awesome, magical) are things that never came to women's minds at all.

As you can see from the figure on the next page,* most women don't seem to be having a whole lot of fun in the luteal phase. And when we look at the content of these not-fun experiences, they don't immediately make sense in the context of implantation and pregnancy. Un-

---

* If you want to do something fun, show this word cloud to your partner or friends and see if they can guess what it is about. I have had about a 90 percent hit rate of people saying something along the lines of "That? Oh, that's PMS," or (my partner's answer) "That? Oh, hell no. I think we both know what that is, but I am too smart a man to say it."

achy acne alienated alone alright **angry** annoyance **annoyed** anti-social anticipation antisocial anxiety **anxious** asthma awful back pain balloon bipolar bitter blah blessed **bloated** boobs so sore **brain fog** breakouts breast pain breast tenderness **calm** calmer challenging changes chill chips chocolate **confused** constantly peeing night and day constipated cozy **cramps** crampy cranky crave-sweets craving sugar **cravings** crushing low **crying** cynical dark dark clothes darker emotions demotivated **depressed** desire to be sedentary desire to be sexually active desolate despair difficult discharge dissociation distracted dizziness drained dread dysfunction easily fatigued eating edgy **emotional** emotional self-regulation empathetic end of the world erratic everyone hates me everything is so loud excited **exhausted** extra meals extreme fatigue false alarms **fatigue** fearful fed up feeling like hangover feeling of dying fever fishy smell flu flu-like food cravings frustrated fuzzy giddy god grim gross grouchy grumpy happy **headache heavy** high energy hip pain histamine reactions home hopeless hormones horny huge **hungry** hungry but no appetite I need chocolate ill tempered impatient impulsive in need of love and acts of care increased appetite inner scream insatiable hunger insomnia intolerant of bs **introspective introverted** intrusive thoughts **irritable** lack of lazy less anxious less hungry less patient lethargic level libido lonely lose patience loss of confidence loss of power lost appetite **low energy** low impact low libido low motivation **low sex drive** make it stop I'm sick of this shit mediocre mellow **migraine** miserable mood **mood swings moody** more trouble sleeping nap **nausea** nauseous neck pain need to clean needy no appetite no sleep normal nostalgic numb occasionally bloated overeating **overwhelmed** painful panic peeing all night physically **pimples** pms poorer sporting performance productive progesterone queasy rage raised heart rate reactive reduced capacity relaxed release relieved resentful resilient rest restless ruminating **sad** scatter brain sedentary **sensitive** shadow short fuse shortness of breath skinny sleepless **sleepy slow** slow runner **sluggish** snacks snacky snappy snuggly **sore** sore boobs sore chest spacey spiritual staring starving **stressed** strong struggle sudden crash suicidal swollen swollen everything tachycardia tampon stash teary tense thankful thick throbbing head **tired** tired but can't sleep trouble sleeping ugly unbalanced uncomfortable undesirable uneventful unfocused ungrounded unhappy uninterested unloved **unmotivated** unsatisfied unsettled unwind upset useless volatile **vulnerable** want comfort **weak** weaker **weepy** why doesn't that person want me withdrawn worry worthlessness

like estrogen and sex, there just isn't an easy-to-see evolutionary story about progesterone and how it makes women feel things that help promote implantation and pregnancy (unless you know something I don't about the pregnancy-boosting benefits of brain fog and sadness). This is the first thing about progesterone and the luteal phase that's a little weird. The experiences we have are virtually indistinguishable from the symptoms of PMS (see table below) and don't seem to have a whole lot to do with supporting the initiation of pregnancy.

The second thing about the luteal phase that's a little weird is that all this misery is orchestrated by a hormone that is routinely praised in the world of neuroscience for its ability to make the brain feel *good*.

. . . ?

Yes, believe it or not, in the weird world of neuroscience, progesterone is known for being a mental health superhero that is supposed to make us feel good. It has anti-inflammatory, neuroprotective, and calm-inducing effects on the brain that are so robust and repeatable that it is currently one of the treatments of choice for traumatic brain injury (decreasing the risk of death by 50 percent in some studies!) and stress-related diseases, such as PTSD and alcohol use disorders.

Here's how it works.

EXPERIENCES COMMONLY NOTED IN WOMEN WITH PMS

AFFECTIVE	COGNITIVE OR PERFORMANCE	SOMATIC
Depression or sadness	Mood swings	Headache
Irritability	Difficulty concentrating	Back pain
Tension	Decreased efficiency	Breast tenderness/ swelling
Anxiety	Confusion	Abdominal cramps/ bloating
Tearfulness/ crying easily	Forgetfulness	General muscle/ joint pain
Restlessness	Prone to accidents	Weight gain
Anger	Temper outbursts	Swelling of extremities
Appetite change		Fatigue
Food cravings		Nausea
Libido change		Insomnia

When progesterone is broken down in the body, it releases an incredibly potent neuroactive steroid (which is nerd-speak for a steroid that affects the excitability of cells in the brain) called allopregnanolone. Allopregnanolone (ALLO for short) has an inhibitory effect on neurons, which means that it makes brain cells less excitable and reactive to things going on in the environment. It does this by stimulating GABA* receptors, which chill out the brain and create an effect similar to what you get from melatonin, massages, meditation, and margaritas. And, as you might expect from a neurosteroid that activates calming pathways in the brain, there is a ton of research demonstrating that progesterone and its calming metabolite ALLO have sedative, anxiolytic (anti-anxiety), anticonvulsant, and neuroprotective effects in the brain. Progesterone and ALLO are like our inner kumbaya,

---

* In case you were wondering, GABA is shorthand for gamma-aminobutyric acid. Nobody calls it this though. It's too much of a mouthful. And I think it sounds too close to *supercalifragilisticexpialidocious* to be taken seriously.

making our brain a more relaxed and sedated version of itself than it is in their absence.

The weird thing about all of this is, of course, that most of us don't feel a whole lot of inner kumbaya in the luteal phase. Sure, women might feel these warm, fuzzy, relaxed states when they're pregnant (which is also a high progesterone state). But within the context of a typical cycle, women's experiences are usually the opposite. The luteal phase is often a time of stress, anxiety, and self-loathing. Progesterone is also the hormone implicated in postpartum depression and PMDD, and is known for worsening symptoms of major depressive disorder (MDD) and other mood and personality disorders.

So, why does a hormone that is known for relaxing the brain and making us feel good make so many of us feel so bad? And why does it also seem to make us feel bloated, tired, foggy brained, snacky, unmotivated, and (in some cases) totally sexually dead inside? What does all that have to do with preparing the body for pregnancy?

The more I began to dig into these questions, the clearer it became that there are two things going on.

The first thing is that a lot of the experiences women report having in the luteal phase are normal and predictable changes that happen as a result of the body transitioning from being all about sex to being all about pregnancy. They just feel disordered because we haven't been given an explanation for why they're happening or what they mean. The result is that women have a lot of experiences that feel like symptoms.

What's the difference, you ask?

Well, when something is wrong with our bodies, we usually experience physical changes that alert us to the fact that there's a problem. These are symptoms. They're smoke that emerges from the fire of pathology. Experiences, on the other hand, are noticeable changes that go on in the body and are expected as part of the body's day-to-day function. Like when we feel hungry because we need food, or we feel tired because we need sleep. Experiences aren't felt as pathological. We understand them to be a meaningful part of the physical wisdom we have inherited from our ancestors to help guide our behavior in ways that ensure our basic needs are met.

Many of the things that go on in the luteal phase are experiences masquerading as symptoms. And because we're not taught what they are, what they mean, and what our bodies need in light of our changing hormonal states, they feel pathological. Like a sign of something wrong.

As you'll learn in the chapters to come, the luteal phase is a time when our bodies experience a lot of physical and psychological changes that no one has told us about. I'm guessing you'll be as surprised as I was to learn that everything ranging from our pain perception to the functional connectivity of our brains looks a little different in the luteal phase than it does in the follicular. And these changes in the body aren't necessarily bad. They just have the tendency to make us feel less than great because we're not taught why they happen or what they mean. These predictable and (as you will learn) functional shifts we have in the luteal phase are only experienced as signs of pathology because we have been taught that our cycles only matter for pregnancy or trying to predict when our periods are going to come.

The second thing going on is that, for many of us, pathology actually gets created in the luteal phase because its needs are routinely ignored. For example, consider the metabolic changes women experience in the luteal phase. Even though all of us have been led to believe that our bodies need the same number of calories every day of the month (all else being equal), this isn't something that's true for women. Our metabolic needs actually increase 7–11 percent in the luteal phase relative to what they are in the follicular phase. So, if you are a woman who eats a 2,000-calorie-a-day diet, this would mean needing roughly 140 additional daily calories to keep the body chugging along at its usual speed in the luteal phase compared to the follicular.

The problem is that most of us aren't told about any of this. Instead, we're given a one-size-fits-all set of guidelines for what our bodies need that we're told applies to us every day of the cycle. And then when we do what we're told (here, not giving your body enough energy in the form of calories), it makes us feel bad. It makes us experience things that most of us are all too familiar with, like food cravings, preoccupation with food, and (when our body finally puts its foot down) binge eating.

Sound familiar?

The food cravings many of us experience in the luteal phase are the result of ignoring the fact that our bodies' needs change in response to our hormonal changes. It's part of what we consider PMS. And it's completely unnecessary. We suffer from food cravings, preoccupation with food, and create an unhealthy, *untrue* narrative about ourselves being lacking in willpower or out of control around food because we are ignoring what our bodies are telling us—*we need more food right now*—because we have all been led to believe that our bodies' needs are one size fits all.

A COUPLE OF WORDS ABOUT THE "PROGESTERONE" IN YOUR HORMONAL BIRTH CONTROL

Of course I had to say a few things about hormonal birth control.

To start with, although hormonal birth control like the pill and hormonal IUD has been great for women in a number of ways, there are a lot of things about these forms of contraception that aren't perfect. For one, they don't contain real-deal, body-identical progesterone. And without real-deal, body-identical progesterone, you lose all the beneficial effects of ALLO that naturally cycling women get. And this is believed to be one of the reasons why hormonal birth control use is linked to an increased risk of anxiety and depression.

The synthetic progesterone in your birth control (called a progestin) is usually synthesized from testosterone (first- through third-generation progestins) or a diuretic called spironolactone (fourth-generation progestins). You can read more about the different types of progestins in birth control and the unique side effect of each in my earlier book, *This Is Your Brain on Birth Control*. For now, it is just worth nothing that these progestins do not offer the calming, mental health benefits of real-deal progesterone. And new research in my lab suggests that progestins also don't offer the same anti-inflammatory effects as real-deal progesterone in response to stress either.

Progesterone and progestins are two very different beasts. And this is important to keep in mind because one of the reasons why progesterone gets such a bad rap is because people are blaming their birth control side effects on progesterone... when there is no progesterone in 99 percent of all hormonal birth control.

It is also worth noting that, because the pill keeps women's hormones consistent across the "cycle" (most birth control has women taking the same dose of hormones every day until they take the sugar pills that kick off their period/withdrawal bleed), most women on the pill don't get PMS. Instead, for pill takers who experience changes in mood across their cycles, these changes usually occur during the week of their period/withdrawal bleed since this is the week that corresponds to their biggest hormonal changes. Natural cyclers get PMS, women on the pill get DMS (during menstrual syndrome).

The problem is that we are not one size fits all. The reason the luteal phase looks like such a confusing mess characterized by PMS-related misery is because we live in a world where women's cyclicity is ignored. So, any changes in what our bodies are doing (particularly if they aren't as fun and pleasurable as those we experience in the fertile window) take on the tint of pathology. Then, when we pretend these changes aren't happening or don't matter, pathology is actually created because our bodies aren't being given what they need to thrive. *This* is why close to 90 percent of us experience PMS. And *this* is why

WHAT WE USUALLY SEE

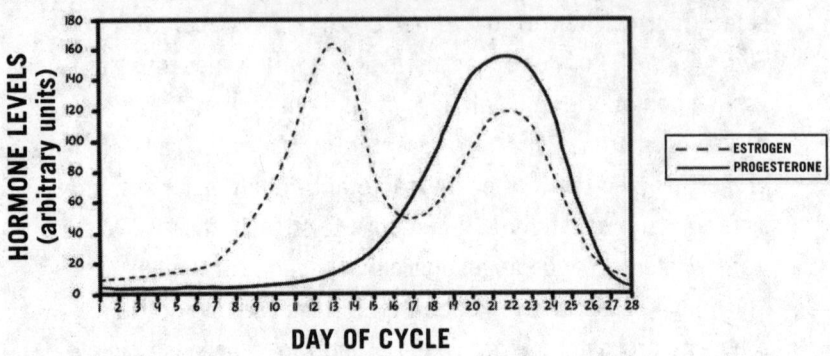

WHAT ACTUALLY GOES ON

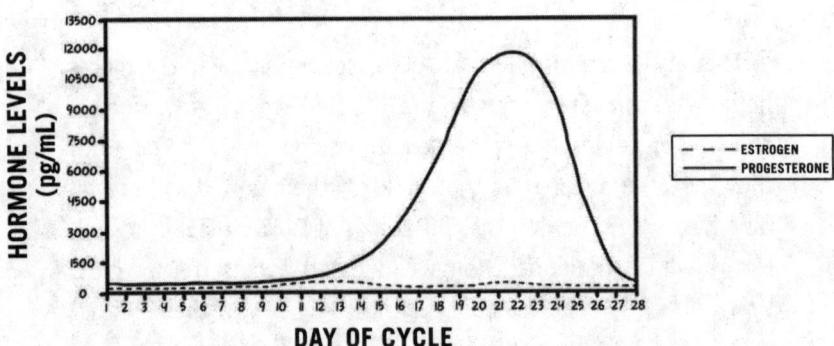

Although the menstrual phase cycle pictures we all see in textbooks and online look like the graph at the top, the scaling of our two hormones is misleading. Generally, estrogen is plotted out in units that are one hundred times smaller than the units used for progesterone. The picture on the bottom is what things would look like if each were plotted using the same units.

there are more than two hundred (!!!) "symptoms" of PMS that have been noted in the research literature. PMS is nothing more than a lazy diagnostic catchall that is used to give women an "explanation" for physical and psychological changes that occur in the luteal phase whether they are occurring on purpose or are a pathology created by ignoring our bodies' needs at this time.

All of this ends here.

We know a lot about estrogen. And for many of us, it's the only hormone we know anything about because progesterone has been treated as an afterthought. Progesterone is so frequently ignored that it was recently left out of a diagram of the menstrual cycle published in a well-respected medical journal. There are nearly three times as many research papers published on the effects of estrogen as there are on the effects of progesterone. And this is true despite the fact that our body produces progesterone at peak levels that are between 25 to 250 times higher than our peak levels of estrogen (see figure on previous page).

Although it is rarely acknowledged, if you are a woman who cycles, you are a beautiful duality. We are a different version of ourselves in the luteal phase than we are in the follicular. When we ignore these differences, we feel fractured and we suffer from PMS. And when we embrace them, we can feel whole.

CHAPTER 4

THE DAWN OF BIKINI SCIENCE

Why everything you thought you knew about "normal" is probably male

Before we dive into the science of who we are and what our bodies need in the luteal phase, I want to first talk about why it's so important to talk freely about the importance of hormonal changes in women's bodies, despite the fact that it might make some of us uncomfortable. I know there's a decent chance that at least some of you are feeling queasy about the idea that our sex hormones matter for anything other than periods and pregnancy. As a woman, I understand fearing that if we speak too loudly about the depth of impact our hormones can have on how we think, feel, and act, this could be used to argue that women are inferior to men and therefore undeserving of equal rights. With consequences of that magnitude, it doesn't feel like something we should be talking about in mixed company, particularly in this post-Roe era, when our political autonomy feels more fragile than ever before in recent history.

The first thing I would like to do is acknowledge this fear. Because it is real and (sadly) warranted. An unfortunate part of being female is that, throughout Western history, our cyclically changing sex hormones have been used as ammunition in arguments about why we shouldn't have the same rights as men. It has been argued that they make us fickle, unpredictable, and less rational than our male counterparts. And as a result, most of us have been taught that the most feminist thing we can do is pretend that our cycles don't matter. It feels scary to talk openly about how our hormonal changes affect us because we have all been led to believe that (a) there is something wrong with hormones affecting feelings, and (b) men are less hormonally volatile than women are.

But, as you'll see, neither of these things are true. Trying to minimize our biological differences from men—rather than removing barriers and liberating us—has been responsible for the complete mismanagement of women in both science and medicine. And it's also how we ended up in a place where the luteal phase became synonymous with a disorder* (PMS).

To start with, let's get comfortable with the idea that our hormones affect how we feel and experience the world. Because they do. There have literally been hundreds of studies published that find that our hormones—including our sex hormones—affect how we feel, our motivational states, the way we think, our ability to learn and remember things, and, of course, our behaviors. And they affect all these things *on purpose*. It's literally their job. Without our hormones changing our feelings and motivational states, there would be no falling in love, escaping from danger, bonding with loved ones, or pushing our limits to win. There would be no *us*. So, there is nothing wrong with—and plenty that's right about—the fact that our hormones affect how we feel and what we do. It's what they're meant to do. Women's hormones affect women. Men's hormones affect men. This is exactly what they should be doing and there is nothing inherently dangerous or weak about it.

The second thing we need to get comfortable with is the fact that our sex hormones cycle. Because despite what sexist half-wits on Reddit might try to tell you, there is nothing about this female-specific factoid that makes us less predictable, rational, or reliable than men. Our hormonal changes across the cycle, rather than being whimsical

---

* Okay, fine: syndrome. But there is a fine line between syndrome and disorder.

and capricious, are predictable to the point of being boring. As I always tell people, if you tell me a woman's age and the first day of her last period, I can give you a pretty accurate read on what's going on with her sex hormones. Our fluctuation between estrogen and progesterone occurs on a very reliable and predictable rhythm. Estrogen is the dominant sex hormone for the first 14-ish days of the cycle. Progesterone is the dominant sex hormone for the second 14-ish days of the cycle. And that's pretty much that. Lather, rinse, repeat. So, women's hormones are cyclical, but not fickle or unpredictable. And anyone who tells you otherwise doesn't know what they're talking about.

Interestingly enough, men's primary sex hormone, testosterone, actually *is* a little unreliable and hard to predict. Not only does it have a cycle (it's highest in the morning and lowest at night . . . which you already knew if you've ever spooned with a man when he's first waking up), it also changes dynamically in response to things going on in the environment. Men's levels of testosterone respond to changes in relationship status, having children, a favorite sports team winning or losing, the loss of a favorite political candidate, having sex, anticipating sex, seeing or interacting with a beautiful woman, and (my own personal favorite) the presence of weapons.

And men's hormonal changes—just like our hormonal changes—have an important impact on how men think, feel, and experience the world. Dynamic changes in men's testosterone levels are part of what prompts men to settle down after getting married and having kids, and to rush the field to knock over goalposts after their favorite team wins. Even though there have been plenty of sexist dipsh*ts throughout the ages who have tried to argue that women aren't cut out for the demands of working, voting, and landownership because our hormones change and men's don't, there is nothing about this idea that is true. Men and women both experience hormonal changes and we are both better off for it.

Although the physical and psychological changes we experience across the cycle have been mischaracterized as something that makes us overly emotional and unpredictable, this idea has absolutely no backing in science. The only reason we've come to perceive these predictable shifts as anything other than completely normal, healthy, or even *desirable* is because our beliefs about "normal" are based on a male standard. But we need to break from this false standard of normalcy and get comfortable with the fact that we differ from men in important ways, including our cycles. Because if we fail to do so—and if those in science and medicine fail to abandon the belief that men and women are more or less interchangeable despite mountains of evidence verifying this isn't true—our needs will continue to go unmet.

The Unbearable Maleness of Being

Although it would be nice to assume that we know as much about our brains and bodies as men know about theirs, we don't. Most of what we know about mental health, physical health, and pretty much anything else involved in the human experience is the result of research conducted on males. This is true whether we're talking about people, nonhuman animals, or even cells (!), making most of our collective wisdom about health, wellness, and personhood something that uses the male body as the standard for what it means to be healthy and normal.

I won't spend too much time going over the reasons that science has excluded females from research since I cover them pretty extensively in my first book. But the short version of the story is that (a) research that includes both sexes takes longer and is more difficult to interpret than research that only includes one (you need to double your sample size, and males and females rarely respond to things the same way), and (b) females are harder to study because you need to account for their hormonal changes, since this is something that could impact research outcomes. Given these challenges, for a very long time scientists did not include any women or female subjects in their research, assuming that male bodies are virtually interchangeable with female bodies (penises, vaginas, and sex hormones notwithstanding).

The problem with this is that the assumption that *as it goes in men, so it must also go in women* is wrong. Like, completely deadass wrong. Because for decades now, research has been documenting a huge range of ways that men and women differ from one another, extending far beyond the size and shape of our reproductive organs. There is sex differentiation all over the place in the body. Our immune systems differ. The processes our bodies use to regulate pain perception differ. Our cardiovascular systems differ. Our brains differ. Our sex hormones differ. The way our bodies metabolize food, drugs, hormones—and everything else our bodies break down for use—differs. Even the way our bodies prefer to capture and kill bacteria differs. (Male bodies use complement opsonization, while female bodies prefer estrogen-driven antibodies, in case you were wondering.)

Biological males and biological females differ down to the cellular and molecular level. Period. End of story.

Despite the mountains of evidence demonstrating that male and female bodies differ in myriad ways beyond the most obvious, science and medicine have routinely tried to downplay these differences. There are a variety of reasons for this, including social desirability (scientists, like everyone else, get squeamish talking too loudly about sex differences for fear of appearing sexist) and the desire to make research easier to conduct. Assuming the sexes differ means needing to develop sex-differentiated research protocols and treatment plans, which is more challenging and time-consuming than just making the decision that one size fits all. So, the position that science and medicine have decided to take is one that assumes that biological sex doesn't matter that much. In the medical world, this approach has been called "bikini medicine" (as in, men and women are indistinguishable with the exception of body parts that get covered by a bikini). So, when applied to research, I call this bikini science.

The problem with taking the bikini approach to science and medicine is that men's and women's responses to things often differ. And failure to contend with this inconvenient fact routinely causes problems that generally have the effect of harming women.

For example, one of the most widely publicized examples of this happened in 1992, when the FDA approved the prescription drug zolpidem (which most of us know by its brand name, Ambien). As with most drugs, research on zolpidem was conducted using samples of mostly male subjects. Also, like most drugs, soon after zolpidem was released into the market, adverse patient reports from women started flooding in. Despite the fact that they were taking a routinely recommended dose of the medication, women were reporting having bad reactions that ranged from prolonged drowsiness to cognitive impairment. Researchers later learned that these effects were the result of the fact that women metabolize the drug much more slowly than men. This means that a woman on a 10 milligram Ambien tablet (the maximum dosage, one that's commonly prescribed) was showing blood levels of the drug consistent with having taken twice that amount. Let me repeat that in case you missed it: *Their blood levels of the drug were consistent with having taken twice that amount.*

Ooops. Sorry, ladies. Our bad.

And the Ambien debacle is far from an isolated incident. Research regularly finds women on the business end of bad side effects, misdiagnoses, and legal standards and safety features that just don't fit our female bodies. Women experience adverse reactions to medication and other forms of medical treatments twice as often as men. Eight out of ten new prescription drugs (80 percent) are regularly pulled from US markets because of unanticipated side effects in women. Women routinely experience diagnostic delays for more than seven hundred different conditions—including heart attack, stroke, cancer, and Parkinson's disease—because of sex-differentiated symptomology.

It's not just medicine that has fallen prey to the false assumption of sex neutrality. The assumption that male = female has harmed us in other ways too. It has resulted in the creation of automobile safety features that are better able to protect men's bodies than women's in car accidents. And it is responsible for the creation of male-biased legal standards that can be harmful to female victims, particularly in the context of sexual violence (for example, the "reasonable person" standard that is used to determine guilt or innocence tends to assume that the reasonable person in question is male, despite men being less likely to see sex crimes as criminal).

Although things have gotten marginally better for women since federal funding agencies started requiring that researchers include (some) females in their research, the problem is far from being solved. This is because the way many researchers are addressing these requirements is perfunctory at best. Women are now being included in research in greater numbers than ever before, but the research is not being done in a way that tests for the effects of biological sex on outcomes being tested.

For example, in one recent analysis of all published papers in the year 2019 in the fields of neuroscience and psychiatry—which are two areas that are *known* to have huge sex differences (it is well documented, for example, that women are diagnosed with anxiety and depression twice as often as men)—only 5 percent of studies tested for biological sex differences on the measured outcomes. *Five percent!* This means that if there were sex differences in whatever was being tested (which, a lot of times, there are), they were completely overlooked because the researchers didn't even test for them.

The whole reason women need to be included in research is because we rarely respond to things in the same way that men do. If women's bodies usually acted the same way as men's bodies in biomedical research, no one would need to study us. But they don't act the same. The only thing this practice of sex inclusion without sex-based data analysis does (besides allowing funding agencies to pat themselves on the back for creating the illusion that they are serving women) is decrease our ability to understand men. So now men and women both lose. And in the weird world of science politics, this is considered progress.

So, the assumption that female and male bodies should not differ from one another when designing research slows the pace of making real progress in science. But it's bad for us in other ways too. Because when we assume that what male bodies do is the standard for what's "normal," it also creates a lens in which everything about us that's different from men becomes problematic. It makes our female-specific traits seem disordered or less than. And you can see evidence of this cultural lens all over the place. You can see it in the sexist hyperbole that calls women fickle, unreliable, and overly emotional because it is assumed that our hormones make us less rational than men. We see it played out in the language we use to describe our cycle-related experiences, which are usually referred to as symptoms (implying that they're an indication of something wrong, instead of experiences that are supposed to happen). And we see it in the way women's periods are treated in cultures across the world. Whether it's relegating women to menstrual huts or making them carry their menstrual products instead of providing them like toilet paper (because, apparently, our periods somehow fall outside the scope of activities that are expected to be managed in public bathrooms), our hormonal changes and our cycles are treated as something outside what is considered part of the normal human experience.

But it's actually worse than you think. Because in addition to putting us at risk medically and creating a cultural lens that pathologizes our differences from men, the assumption that women are just like men with different reproductive organs has also been foundational in shaping the agreed-upon procedures for dealing with women's cycles in research. And it is one that all but guarantees that women won't understand how their brains and bodies work in the luteal phase.

Making Females Less Female

Although it took scientists a long time to recognize that women and female subjects needed to be included in research, once they did, they had to figure out how to deal with our differences from men. And because the guiding assumption in science has been that women are like men plus some lady hormones, this meant that researchers had to figure out how to deal with our cycles.

Now, there are a couple of ways that scientists could have chosen to deal with our hormonal changes, each of which is guided by a slightly different set of assumptions about what hormones do and how they affect our bodies. The first possible solution is testing women in the follicular phase *and* the luteal phase of the cycle. This is a solution guided by the assumption that women's two primary sex hormones are each an integral part of who women are and will impact how their bodies respond to things (whether it is an experimental manipulation, a new therapy or drug, or anything else). And this is also a solution that recognizes that women's changing sex hormones are part of what normal looks like for women: that there are two halves to a woman's whole, meaning that it is necessary to test them twice to get a complete picture of how their brains and bodies react to anything.

The second possible solution is to include women in research during points in the cycle when their sex hormones are *low*. That is, rather than measuring how women's bodies respond to treatments in both the luteal and follicular phases, this solution minimizes the impact of women's hormones on research outcomes by excluding women from research when their hormone levels are high. The assumption guiding this solution is that male equals normal and female hormones interfere with—rather than are a part of—what normal looks like for half of the population.

Can you guess which of these two solutions the world of science landed on to account for women's changing sex hormones?

That's right, science chose the latter solution. And, as a result, the current gold standard procedure for including women and other female subjects in biomedical research as of this writing (2025) is one that specifies that women should be included in research only during days in the cycle in which levels of sex hormones are *low*. When females are at their least female.

When testing on human subjects like we do in my research lab, this means testing women only on Days 3 through 7 of the cycle. At this time, levels of estradiol are far lower than they are when they approach their ovulatory peak. And progesterone levels are practically nonexistent. Measuring all women during this narrow time frame ensures that all the women in the study are relatively similar to one another hormonally since they are all in the same cycle phase. It also ensures that the women in the study are maximally similar to men since their levels of female-specific sex hormones are relatively low. And for research in nonhuman animals, the way sex hormones are dealt with is even worse. Researchers will often remove female animals' ovaries to ensure that they don't release sex hormones at all. Doing research in ways that try to artificially minimize female animals' differences from male animals makes research results less messy and makes causal conclusions easier to come by, but it ensures that we will never understand women's bodies.

Having very low levels of sex hormones isn't something that's typical for women. We are hormonal creatures. Researchers estimate that we spend less than 20 percent (!) of our cycle in a hormonal state similar to the one we're usually tested in. Because of this, knowing how we respond to a specific drug or therapy when hormone levels are low won't necessarily provide any insight into how our bodies will respond the other twenty-two-plus days of the cycle when our hormone levels are *high*.

This scientific choice means that our understanding of the way women's bodies respond to everything—ranging from stress and exercise to prescription drugs and vaccines—is incomplete, particularly in the luteal phase. And this is an important omission because the way our bodies respond to things can differ—sometimes in pretty dramatic ways—depending on the cycle phase in which they're measured.

In one study, for example, researchers found that the relationship between our levels of the stress hormone cortisol and the amount of distress we feel in response to a stressful event does a complete 180 across the cycle. You can see the results for yourself in the figures below. For women in the estrogenic follicular phase, cortisol levels were negatively related to how bad women felt in response to a stressful event (consistent with the idea that cortisol helps resolve stress). For women in the progestogenic luteal phase, however, the opposite

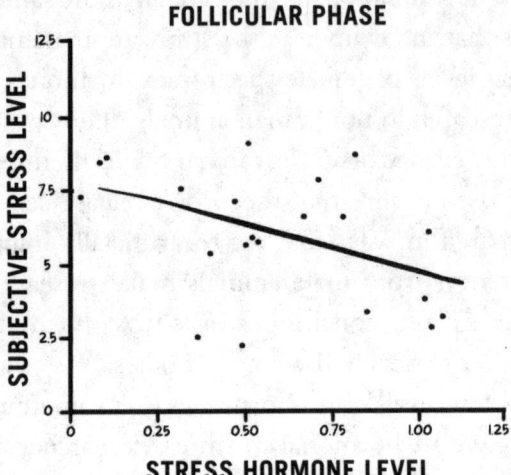

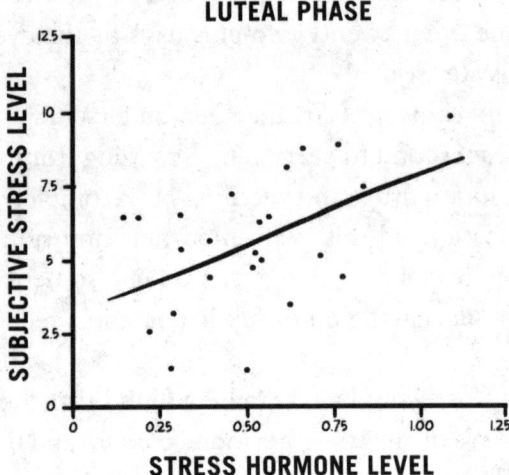

was found. For these women, the ones who felt the worst were those whose cortisol levels were highest.

If the researchers had only looked at the relationship between cortisol and stress in the follicular phase (the current gold standard for doing research in women), the headline would read "Cortisol Improves Women's Subjective Stress." And if women went to their doctor's office with reports of feeling anxious while taking a medication that stimulates cortisol receptors (for example, if they were on a glucocorticoid medication, such as hydrocortisone or dexamethasone), their doctor would tell them that they have no idea why that is happening. And that, if anything, they should actually be feeling less anxious in response to their medication. *Perhaps the answer is a higher dose?*

And if the researchers failed to divide women based on their cycle phase at all and simply looked at the relationship between stress hormones and stress level in all women at once, the results would have looked like the figure below. And the headline would have read "No Relationship Between Cortisol and Women's Subjective Stress." Then women would again be led to feel like they are crazy for having their levels of anxiety change in response to a medication whose impact on anxiety levels was masked by the fact that researchers never bothered to look at cycle phase.

Although it is an inconvenient truth for science and medicine to need to contend with, female sex hormones are an integral part of

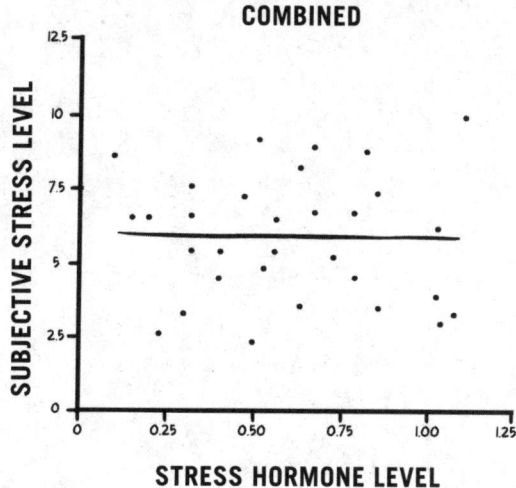

female normal. And female normal has two halves. And when we're only given half of the story of ourselves, everything that goes on in the last two weeks can feel like pathology. There is no way to truly understand women—whether it's our mental health, our responses to medication, or our energy and activity needs—without understanding who we are and what our bodies need in the season of each of our primary sex hormones.

The one-size-fits-all approach to understanding humans doesn't work for women. It makes us feel like there's something about us that's broken. And most of us have no choice but to believe this narrative is true because we haven't ever been told what it looks like when things are going *right*.

I have spent the last several years of my life working to address this huge gap in our self-understanding, piecing together answers from the research literature to help you understand who you are and what your body needs in the luteal phase. So, let's dive in to everything I have learned. You might find answers to your own cycle-related concerns.

PART II

RECLAIMING FEMALE

Rethinking PMS and
Embracing Hormonal Change

CHAPTER 5

UNDERSTANDING THE LUTEAL PHASE

*Progesterone creates unique physical
and psychological needs*

You know by now that your body has two biologically distinct ways of being. There is the estrogen version of you, which is sexy, fun, and talked about nonstop on TikTok videos. And then there is the progesterone version of you,* which no one ever talks about. The next chapters of the book are designed to help introduce you to the two weeks in the cycle that science, medicine, and even social media usually ignore.

And there's a lot to learn. As you'll see, the luteal phase is a time of greater metabolic demand, greater exposure to hormonal changes, and greater vulnerability to threats of all sorts compared to the follicular phase. And these changes are each the result of the fact that our bodies are preparing for the possibility of pregnancy, which requires a lot of workarounds. Our body has to change the rules it uses for everything from danger detection to pathogen neutralization, because

---

* When I say estrogen-you and progesterone-you, note that this is shorthand for which of our two primary sex hormones is dominant at that particular cycle phase. But don't take this too literally. Progesterone-you, for example, is also releasing estrogen.

many of the rules in the follicular phase don't work for a body preparing for pregnancy. So even though most of the cultural conversation about progesterone and the luteal phase is about how awful we feel, at the heart of many of these awful feelings is a brilliantly designed system managing the biological realities of possible pregnancy.

The Biological Realities of Being a Human Female in the Luteal Phase

As a reminder, the luteal phase of the cycle gets kicked off after ovulation. This is when progesterone begins being released from that temporary endocrine structure formed in the just-vacated egg follicle. Progesterone release serves as the body's cue to begin shifting gears from being all about sex and attraction to being all about supporting a pregnancy. And this shift takes a ton of work. The whole body has to work together to modify its physical and psychological landscape to accommodate the growth of another human being for nine months. For example, the circulatory system has to allow the blood supply to be shared with a developing fetus; the immune system has to become tolerant of foreign bodies to allow embryonic implantation; and the brain has to shift our motivational states in ways that increase our interest in doing things that encourage healthy pregnancies (e.g., eating, napping) and decrease our interest in things that don't (e.g., working eighteen-hour days, bungee jumping). And this is just a short list. There is a whole lot of cellular switch flipping and gear shifting that needs to go on to accommodate growing a brand-new human being. The net effect of all this is that the luteal phase is biologically distinct from the follicular phase. Here are just a few of the biological realities that our bodies are confronted with at this time that make it unique.

Biological Reality Number 1: The luteal phase is a time of huge hormonal changes. The first thing that we need to appreciate about the luteal phase is that there is a lot more going on with our sex hormones at this time than there is during the follicular phase. Like, a *lot* more. To contextualize this for you, the biggest hormone change that happens in the follicular phase is the estrogen surge that precedes ovulation. At this time, estrogen levels increase to levels three to ten times higher than where they are in the early follicular phase. This is a 200–900 percent (!) increase in hormone levels, which I think you'd agree is pretty substantial, but it's got nothing on the luteal phase.

In the luteal phase, progesterone levels increase to peak levels that are around twenty-five times higher than what they are in the follicular phase. This means that they're about 2,400 percent (!) higher than what they were right after ovulation. And then they decrease by this same magnitude. And remember: Progesterone peaks at concentrations that are up to 250 times higher than peak concentrations of estrogen, making this a lot of hormonal change in a short period of time. And this is just half of it. Because in addition to these big swings in progesterone that we get in the luteal phase, we also have a second rise and fall of estrogen at this time. Although the latter isn't as substantial as the one we have before ovulation, it's far from insignificant. (See the drawing of the cycle on page 36 for a visual reminder). Navigating these changes gracefully requires a lot of cellular plasticity.

For example, remember when we talked about how progesterone releases a calming neurosteroid called ALLO when it is broken down in the body? And how it activates our GABA receptors, producing calming effects in the brain? Well, when levels of progesterone rise and fall in the cycle, this also means rising and falling levels of ALLO. If our brain's GABA receptors are able to adapt to these changes without incident, they might not feel that noticeable. But for women whose GABA receptors are slower to make the necessary adjustments, it can create serious problems with mood and stress regulation.

Biological Reality Number 2: The luteal phase is a time when our immunological defenses are down. During the luteal phase, our body taps the brakes on the immune system so that it doesn't go on a search-and-destroy mission every time it gets a whiff of DNA that doesn't belong to itself. Because if it did, embryos would never have a shot at implantation. Although the presence of non-self-DNA is one of the hallmarks of immunological bad guys like bacteria, parasites, and viruses (which our immune system is supposed to kill), it is also a feature of sperm, embryos, and fetuses (which they are not). So, one of progesterone's jobs in the luteal phase is to suppress our immune system to prevent our bodies from waging an all-out immunological war every time a fertilized egg makes an appearance in the endometrium and tries to hack into our blood supply.

On the bright side, tapping the brakes on the immune system has a wonderfully anti-inflammatory effect in the body (more about this in chapter 9). But the darker side is that it can make us more susceptible to illness and infection in the luteal phase than we are in the follicular. This is why the severity of many infectious diseases increase during pregnancy. Pregnancy is a high progesterone state, and because of this we're more vulnerable to illnesses that rely on inflammatory activity for controlling their spread in the body.

Biological Reality Number 3: Progesterone makes you hotter. Literally. Your basal body temperature (BBT) rises almost a full degree[*] Fahrenheit in the luteal phase compared to what it is in the follicular. This change is usually evident a day or so after ovulation and then stays with us until the end of the luteal phase, when our periods start.[†] Having a higher temperature makes it harder for bacteria and viruses to survive, which is one of the ways our bodies help keep us from getting sick when our immunological pants are down. (This is also why we get fevers; germs hate heat.) Although this biological reality isn't terribly consequential in terms of how any of us experience the world (beyond making us sweatier during our workouts and more inclined to shed the extra blanket at night[‡]), it has the down-

---

[*] Although one recent study found average temperature increases are lower (clocking in at only 0.33 degree Fahrenheit higher) when measured using wearable tech like the Oura Ring or Apple Watch. Just FYI, if you measure your BBT with wearables like I do.

[†] Fun fact: If BBT does not return to baseline after fourteen days (when the luteal phase typically ends), this can be an early indication of pregnancy.

[‡] Interestingly enough, research finds that our progestogenic temperature increase is more noticeable at night than during the day. So if you heat up like a furnace at

stream effect of increasing our resting metabolic rate, which brings us to biological reality number 4 . . .

Biological Reality Number 4: Your energy needs are higher in the luteal phase than they are in the follicular. There's a reason you feel so snacky in the last two weeks of the cycle. I touched on this briefly in chapter 3, but here it is again: We burn somewhere between 7–11 percent more calories in the luteal phase than the follicular. This means we need more (high-quality) food to fuel ourselves at this time. Our energy burn increases because the changes in core body temperature—as well as the other changes our body has to make to prepare for pregnancy—are metabolically expensive. They require a lot of fuel. Our body is a metabolic powerhouse in the luteal phase, burning through energy, nutrients, and amino acids in ways that increase our food intake needs in the last two weeks of the cycle.

Biological Reality Number 5: You have fewer resources to dedicate to everything that isn't pregnancy preparation. One theme that you have undoubtedly picked up on here is that fueling the transformation of your body from a fun, flirty, sex kitten into the sort of matronly vessel that can grow, protect, and nurture new life is a metabolically costly affair. It requires a ton of energy, nutrients, and other resources that can become depleted each month as the body works to fuel the demanding work of pregnancy preparation.

To give you an idea of what this actually looks like, in one study, researchers measured levels of different types of amino acids and lipids in women's blood and urine at five different points across the menstrual cycle (determined by hormone measures and menstrual data). The five phases were: menstrual, follicular, periovulatory (i.e., the fertile window), luteal, and premenstrual. On the next page, you can see the concentrations of the different amino acid and lipid metabolites found in women's fluids at the different times in their cycles. Solid bars are metabolites that are depleted, with darker coloration mean-

---

night like I do in the luteal phase, you are far from alone. Pro tip: I find that I sleep a lot better when I lower the thermostat an extra degree during the luteal phase to accommodate my higher temperature. It works every time.

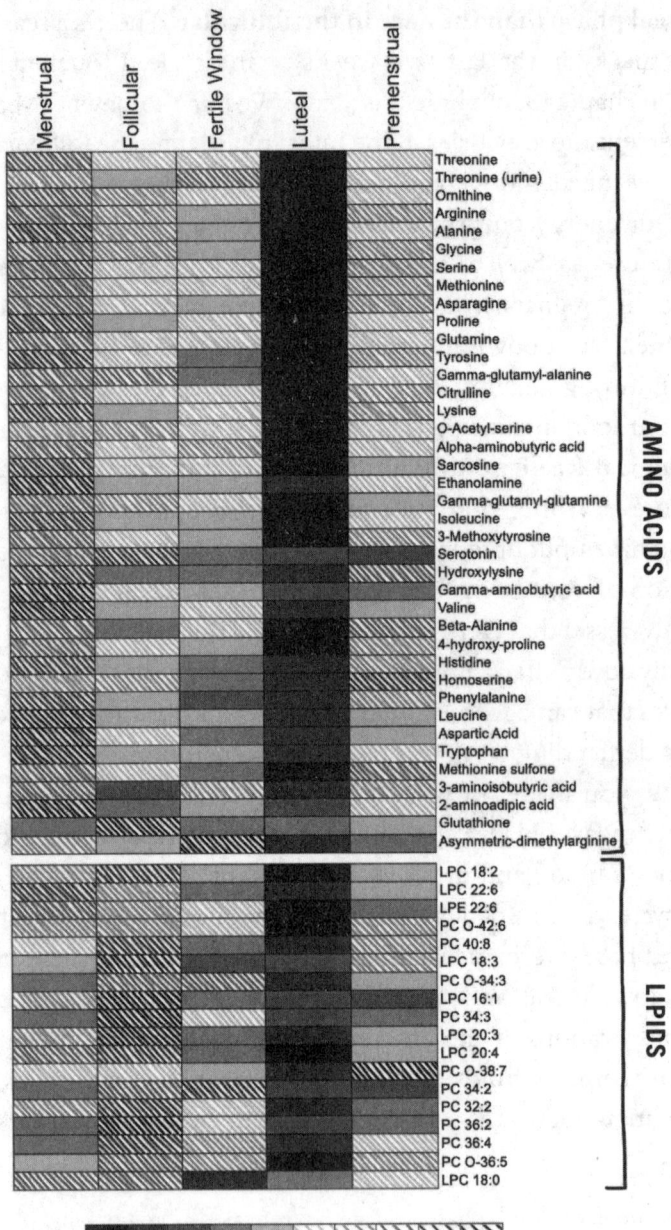

ing greater depletion. Bars with hatch marks are metabolites that are replenished, with darker coloration meaning greater replenishment.

As you can see, the luteal phase—particularly at its peak, when the body is in full-steam-ahead pregnancy-preparation mode—is a time in which our metabolic resources are very much in demand, depleting resources that our body uses for essential functions like energy production, protein and neurotransmitter synthesis, immune function, and antioxidant function.

And it's not just our nutrients that get depleted; our ability to be resilient to—and recover from—stress is also lower in the luteal phase than in the follicular phase. If you are someone who wears a smart watch, WHOOP band, or Oura Ring, you may have noticed this already. Women's recovery scores tend to be lower[*] in the luteal phase than the follicular because our body is working harder and needs more time in recovery than it does in the follicular phase.

Biological Reality Number 6: The luteal phase is a time in which the cost of social abandonment—whether by our friends, families, or romantic partners—is higher than it is in the follicular. Although the cost of being abandoned by the people we rely on for love, care, help, and companionship is always high, there is no time in a woman's life when these costs are higher than they are during pregnancy or when caring for young children. This is true now—whether you want this to be true or not, single mothers and children of single mothers tend to fare less well than partnered women and their children on just about every metric a person might measure—and was even more true for our female ancestors. They didn't have access to security systems, food delivery, and daycare centers to help keep everyone safe, fed, and cared for in the absence of a partner. For most of human history, if you were a woman—especially one who

---

[*] I, for one, have noticed that I can abuse my body in any number of ways in the follicular phase—whether it's not getting enough sleep, getting too much exercise, or having cocktails with dinner—and still have fairly amazing recovery and feel good. When I do any of these things in the luteal phase, though, my recovery is trash and I feel like it too.

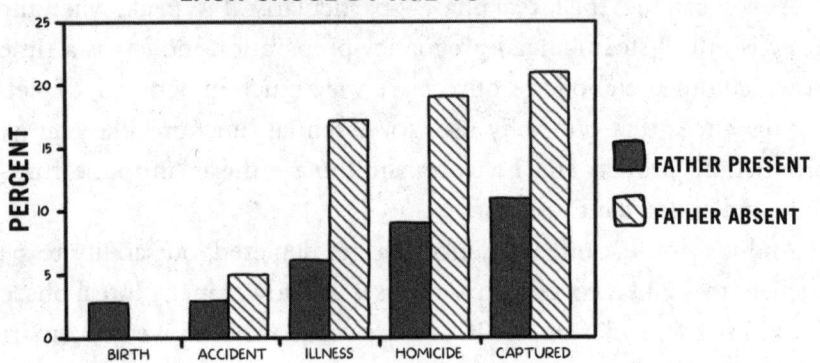

was pregnant or had children—the survival chances for you and your children were far, *far* lower if you didn't have a partner or community around to help out.

For example, in one study conducted on the Aché,* who are a small Indigenous population of hunter-gatherers living in eastern Paraguay, researchers were interested in looking at the degree to which paternal involvement played a role in the survival of children among those living in the types of hunter-gatherer groups that our ancestors spent most of their history. As you can see from the figure above, children without fathers were more likely to die of every cause recorded with the exception of childbirth. This suggests that children of single mothers likely didn't fare well in our ancestral environments . . . and their mothers probably didn't fare very well either.

Although the children of unpartnered women in industrialized nations have a much better chance of survival than the children of unpartnered Aché women (and the risk of our children being captured is inarguably lower across the board . . . at least one would hope), they still fare worse than their peers from two-parent households. Throughout history and now, women have benefited from investments made by their partners, families, and communities to help with

---

* Pronounced "Ah-chay" in case you ever need to say it out loud.

the demanding job of raising our unusually needy offspring. There's a reason they say "it takes a village." And because the luteal phase is all about preparing for pregnancy, it is a time when we become more sensitive to the risk of losing our partners and our village because this is precisely when we need them most.

Biological Reality Number 7: The luteal phase is a time of greater physical vulnerability compared to the follicular. This one is pretty obvious, but worth mentioning. Women are more physically vulnerable in the luteal phase than the follicular because of the whole you-might-be-pregnant, baby-on-board thing. This means that if you are to get injured during this time, you're not just injuring yourself. You're potentially injuring your unborn child too.

But also there are other changes going on in our bodies at this time that make injuries more costly. For example, progesterone (and its sidekick hormone, relaxin) loosens our joints and tendons in ways that are great for pregnancy and childbirth but may increase our risk of certain sports injuries. To make matters worse, our ability to heal from injuries may be slower at this time. This is because of the immunological suppression discussed above and also because progesterone is catabolic (meaning it likes to break things down instead of building them up). This can make it harder for injured tissue to get repaired, making our "normal" activities riskier than they are in the follicular phase.

Biological Reality Number 8: The luteal phase is a time when sex is no longer going to result in pregnancy. This is also obvious, but again worth mentioning. An egg can only survive unfertilized in the reproductive tract for twenty-four hours post-release. This means that luteal-phase sex is a reproductive dead end. And because the evolutionary process rewards behaviors that promote successful reproduction, this means that the evolutionary balance of risks and rewards from sex changes in the luteal phase in ways that can mean bad news for our sexual desire.

And this is just the beginning. As you'll see, progesterone unleashes a host of physical and psychological changes in the body that have a cascading impact on everything ranging from our moods, motivational states, sexual desire, pain perception, vulnerability to addiction, ability to put on muscle mass, and the list goes on. In the next several chapters, we are going to begin to unearth who that version of ourselves is. And we'll get this started by talking about changes in mood. Because one of the most commonly reported experiences that women have in the luteal phase is that it can feel like an emotional roller coaster. So let's dive in and see what we can do to smooth the ride.

CHAPTER 6

IS THERE A METHOD TO YOUR MADNESS?

The upside to feeling down

Although there are a lot of cool and interesting ways that our brains and bodies rewire themselves during the luteal phase (I think the changes in metabolism and sexual desire are particularly spicy), one of the most noticeable changes we experience during this phase in the cycle is that our moods change . . . and not in a way that most of us appreciate. As we saw in our depressingly gray premenstrual mood map in chapter 1, most women have the experience of feeling somewhat less happy and positive in the luteal phase than they do in the follicular.

Consider the experiences of Christina* and Maya, who each undergo a different version of mood changes in the luteal phase.

Christina is a thirty-seven-year-old married mother of two. This is what she had to say: "My mood changes weren't that bad until my first child was born. Then the wheels came off completely. It's like, I'd be looking forward to plans with my friends and be happy and productive at work and then . . . *bam*. About ten to fourteen days before my period, my mood would turn on a dime. It's like I couldn't

---

* All women described here and throughout the book are fictional composite characters made up using elements from multiple women's real stories (along with some made-up details to personify the characters).

even recognize myself. I'd be crying, screaming that nobody understands. . . . I just felt so alone. I'd go to work, take care of my family, and then basically lock myself up in the bedroom for the rest of the day to cry and feel sorry for myself. I took Prozac for two years to help manage, but it made me feel like a zombie, so I quit. Now . . . well . . . I am feeling better with therapy, but my mood is still a struggle each month."

Maya is a twenty-nine-year-old executive with a demanding schedule and a live-in boyfriend. Her mood changes were less severe than Christina's and were more about feeling tired, unmotivated, and sensitive than sad: "My mood in the luteal phase? Where do I start? I feel like I have no motivation to do anything. I just feel *blah* and like I can't talk myself into being as productive as I want. And I hate how I am with my boyfriend. It feels like he can't do anything right. If he loads the dishwasher wrong or forgets to pick up our dry cleaning, not only does it annoy me more than normal, it feels like a referendum on our relationship. It's like *you would load the dishwasher correctly if you cared more about me*, which I recognize is ridiculous, but it feels real in the moment."

Let's unpack the science behind these mood changes. As you will see, the reasons behind the emotional and motivational changes that many of us go through in the luteal phase are as complex as we are. And the way that each of us experiences our mood changes is unique. We'll start with the deep, evolutionary wisdom of our changing psychological weather forecast in the luteal phase and see that clouds, while expected, don't always need to lead to rain.

The Upside to Feeling Down

Before I get into the science of luteal-phase mood changes, let me assure you that they are incredibly common. Research shows that women tend to feel tired, sluggish, unmotivated, and socially withdrawn in the luteal phase. We become less interested in engaging with the outside world, more internally focused, and don't really feel like having to play nicely in the sandbox with others. And this happens not just because we've all had the sexist premenstrual = bad equation embedded into our unconscious. Even female baboons—whose sexist cultural narratives are far less sophisticated than ours—want to be alone during the luteal phase. Research finds that they're more likely to spend time alone in trees than on the ground socializing with peers during the luteal phase (with the pattern reversed in the follicular).

Although these feelings aren't a whole lot of fun, it turns out that feeling tired, sluggish, and socially withdrawn are things that our bodies do on purpose. It's the result of our body shifting its energy away from external pursuits (attraction! sex!) toward the very internal, very costly pursuit of pregnancy preparation in response to progesterone release. Progesterone gets our brains to shift gears using a couple of clever tricks that can make us feel more internal, anxious, and less motivated to GSD* than we are in the follicular phase.

So let's talk about them.

The first way that progesterone gets us to shift our energy inward is through the release of allopregnanolone (ALLO). In case you don't remember this neurosteroid from chapter 3 (see page 31), it is that wondrously calming metabolite that gets released when our bodies break down progesterone. This means that any time progesterone levels increase (*hellllloooo, luteal phase*), it will soon be followed by a rise in ALLO. This has a pretty intense chill-out effect on the brain because ALLO stimulates our brain's GABA receptors, which slow down the brain and make it less reactive to things. It makes us a sleepier, less energetic, and more inward-focused version of ourselves. These changes can make us feel good in some ways (think how cozy it feels when we're snuggled up on the couch with a good book or after a hot bath or massage). But it can also make us feel less energetic and more subdued. For some women, this shift can register on the emotional radar screen as low-key sadness.

Progesterone also modulates hormone sensitivity and neurotransmission in ways that make effort more effortful, pleasurable less

---

* Get sh*t done.

pleasurable, and rewards* less rewarding. This is a great strategy for conserving energy and staying safe (when nothing seems worth doing or having, you aren't going to work very hard or put yourself in harm's way to get it) but can add to the general feeling of unmotivated malaise that many women experience in the luteal phase.

Here's how it works.

Normally, when our brain spots something "wantable"—whether it's a promotion at work, a hot guy, or those gorgeous black ballet flats that keep popping up on your social feed—our pleasure pathways get activated and dopamine gets released. It creates a neurobiological cascade that feels all *"Ooooh, I want that!"* and *"Give me more!"* These feelings will then motivate whatever effort is necessary to make our wanting a reality. And once we get whatever it is that we've been working for, our brain gets rewarded for its efforts with the experience of pleasure, which is created from dopamine, serotonin, and lots of beautiful neural fireworks in the nucleus accumbens (which is your brain's reward hub).

When progesterone is on the scene, though, it's like the fun police arrived and dimmed the lights on the party. Not only does progesterone turn down the volume on pleasure (which makes the things we like less enjoyable), it also decreases their reward value, which makes them less desirable, so we want them less.† So sex feels less sexy, hang-

---

* Not all of them, mind you. Just many. An exception to this is food rewards. We find food more rewarding in the luteal than follicular phase. Another one that might be an exception is sleep. It's easy to imagine that our brain would find sleep and resting more rewarding in the luteal phase.

† In case you were wondering, pleasure and reward are created by closely related but distinct processes in the brain. Pleasure is the same as liking. It is the subjective feeling of pleasure or euphoria that comes from an enjoyable activity. Reward, on the other hand, refers to the motivational component associated with a reward or experience. It's about wanting. And just to give you an example of how these two things are separate from each other, consider all the times you've found yourself eating an addictive but not terribly enjoyable food. I had this experience myself recently when I was at the movies and found myself eating my son's movie popcorn. It didn't taste good (it was stale!), but I kept wanting to eat it because it was activating the reward circuits in my brain.

ing out with our friends feels less friendtastic, and many of the other things that we usually enjoy and want to do don't seem as enjoyable or worth doing in the luteal phase than they seem when we're outside of it.

Progesterone shifts our motivational priorities in this way to help promote pregnancy preparation. It's all part of the brain's master plan to help get your genes into the next generation. Although distorting reality in this way may seem an odd thing for our brain to do, turning the volume up and down on rewards is one of the brain's oldest tricks when it comes to influencing behavior. When there is something our brain wants us to do, it makes it seem more pleasurable and rewarding (this is why sex hits differently in the fertile window*). And when there's something that our brain wants us to avoid, it does the opposite (this is why it feels bad to hurt ourselves or others). Pleasure = yes, I'll do it, even if it requires effort. Pain = no way am I doing that sh*t again. So, when something that normally seems exciting and enticing suddenly seems less so, we usually think, *Meh, maybe next time.*

That our brains turn down the volume on both pleasure and wanting is the reason that so many women feel unmotivated and blah during the luteal phase. Not getting the type of pleasure we expect to get out of things we enjoy is a hallmark of depression and even experiencing it temporarily and in a mild form isn't much fun. It can make the world feel a little gray and uninteresting, which is—unfortunately—pretty common during the luteal phase.

Progesterone can change our motivational landscape in ways that are energy conserving but can make us feel like we are square in the middle of *Blahsville*. In a lot of ways, this would be bad enough on its own (especially when it's contrasted with how amazing and energetic we feel in the fertile window). But as luck would have it, this is just the warm-up act, because progesterone also changes our perception in ways that can make us more inclined to look for alligators in mud puddles . . . which can cause its own set of problems with our mood.

---

* We both know this is true.

Threat Sensitivity in the Season of Progesterone

Before we dive headfirst into the ways that progesterone can distort our perception of reality (but functionally! and on purpose!), we need to talk a little about perception. The way we interpret the world around us is filled with a lot of guesswork rather than objectivity. Most of the time, when we think we know why things happen and what they mean, they are actually just educated guesses our brains make based on the best evidence available at the time. For example, if we're trying to figure out whether our new coworker likes us, we'll look at whatever evidence we have that might bear on this question and draw conclusions accordingly. If she goes out of her way to talk to us, gives us compliments, and offers us help on projects, we might assume she likes us. Conversely, if it seems like she goes out of her way to avoid us, never returns favors, and didn't invite us to her holiday party, we will probably assume she doesn't. Whatever guess we make, it is unlikely that we will ever know with 100 percent certainty whether it's right or wrong. We just make the best guess we can based on the information we have available, assume it's right, and hope for the best.

When it comes to making guesses about things that might pose a threat to us—like the dangerousness of a sketchy stranger or the edibility of sketchy leftovers—our brains like to err on the side of assuming danger. We intentionally don't give the same weight to evidence suggesting that something is safe as we do to evidence suggesting that something is dangerous because it's almost always better to be safe than sorry. The cost of assuming that something is safe when it's actually dangerous could result in death, injury, or worse, whereas the cost of assuming that something is dangerous when it's actually safe is usually far less serious. The smoke detector at your house works the same way. They are wired to err on the side of danger. Sounding the alarm every time you make a pizza is a far lesser sin than failing to alarm and missing an actual fire.

Another interesting thing about the way our brains work is that our tendency to err on the side of danger is highly sensitive to context. Our sensitivity to danger gets turned up and down depending on just how sorry we would be if we failed to be safe. When we're in a more vulnerable state, our brain lowers the bar for the type of things that will set off alarm bells as potential threats. When we're less vulnerable, it does the opposite. This is why men are less afraid of walking alone at night than women. And also why Chihuahuas spook more easily than pit bulls. Being in a vulnerable state puts the brain on high alert, and even the most innocuous threats can seem like a real danger.

THIS IS YOUR MOOD ON TESTOSTERONE

One of the cooler things I have learned about hormones in recent years is that testosterone is protective against anxiety. Testosterone—in addition to all the other things it does (*hello, libido*)—serves as one of the indexes of our body's vulnerability to physical threats. We can be more calm and relaxed when testosterone levels are high than when testosterone levels are low, because it provides an internal cue to our ability to protect ourselves. Our bodies produce more testosterone when we are healthy and strong than they do when they are weak or sick. Extra vigilance isn't necessary when testosterone levels are high because we are in good enough shape to have our own backs.

This means that we can help support our mental health (especially if we suffer from anxiety and depression) by supporting healthy testosterone levels. We can do this with resistance training (building muscle is excellent for supporting testosterone production and has other positive mental health benefits as well), getting enough high-quality sleep (great for all of our hormones), and keeping a healthy body weight (body fat releases aromatase, which converts testosterone into estrogen).

There are few times in women's lives when they are more vulnerable to everything than when they are pregnant or preparing for pregnancy. It would make sense then that progesterone lowers the bar on how certain the brain has to be that something is actually a threat before it sets off alarm bells. Although it's always better to be safe than sorry with threats, the benefits of heightened vigilance are particularly high when women are pregnant. Progesterone changes how our brains process information in ways that can make everything more likely to take on a patina of danger than it does in the follicular phase.

Consistent with this idea, research finds that women in romantic relationships exhibit heightened abandonment fears in the luteal phase compared to the follicular. This happens because progesterone heightens sensitivity to even the subtlest signs of threat in our relationships because the cost of having our partner leave when pregnant is so high that it's worth the cost of a little extra vigilance. This is why it might not feel like a big deal to us if our partner has to stay late at work when we're in the first two weeks of our cycle . . . but it might set off alarm bells during weeks three and four. It's also why women like Maya, whom we met at the beginning of our chapter, are more likely to see subtle slights—like the failure to load the dishwasher correctly—as harbingers of danger in the relationship.

And it's not just our romantic partners who can set off our alarm bells. Research finds that women are more sensitive to social threats of all sorts in the luteal phase, which is likely why so many women report wanting to spend more time alone in the luteal phase than follicular. For example, research finds that when progesterone levels are high, women are more likely to perceive negative emotions in the faces of people making neutral expressions than they are when progesterone levels are low. Women also perceive others' negative emotions as being more intense when progesterone is high than when it is low. Specifically, researchers found that women perceived angry or sad faces as being angrier or sadder than they believed them to be when progesterone was low.

These changes are guided by adjustments in how our brain does business in response to progesterone release. Progesterone increases the reactivity of the amygdala (our brain's built-in security system), lowering the bar on how threating something has to appear before we sound the alarm bells. It also causes changes in the brain's intrinsic connectivity that correspond to increased vigilance to threat. For example, it increases the number of connections between the amygdala and other parts of the brain, which means that our brain's security system is able to gather input from and send output to a greater variety of brain regions in the luteal phase than the follicular.

So, if you find yourself feeling a little more anxious and . . . shall we say . . . *emotionally responsive* to signs of threat in the luteal phase, you are far from alone. It is incredibly common for women to feel more negatively charged in the luteal phase. I've heard women describe this shift in responsiveness to feeling like their blinders have come off and they can finally see things clearly. Like, suddenly they're aware of all the terrible injustices they'd somehow foolishly missed. In a lot of ways, we're right about this, because our brain actually *is* more attuned to subtle signs of threat in the luteal phase than the follicular. But it's also true (and I find this useful to keep in mind when I'm having a luteal-phase moment and feel like everyone hates me) that this greater attunement doesn't increase our *accuracy* at detecting threats. It just means that we'll be less likely to miss a threat should one occur. Feelings are not facts. And the experiences that many of us have in the luteal phase are a good reminder of this.

Although our luteal-phase mood changes can feel difficult, there is wisdom in our discomfort. It increases our ability to detect and avoid possible sources of harm at a time when we're most vulnerable to them. Unpleasant feelings serve an important function in the body (see list on the next page). And even though it's no fun to feel bad, it's better than the alternative. Lacking an internal barometer that screams "Stop doing that, you fool!!" when you're doing things that are harmful is a recipe for disaster.

The changes we experience across the cycle have helped our successful ancestors navigate the demands and vulnerabilities inherent in pregnancy. Our emotional changes across the cycle are a manifes-

EMOTIONAL CHANGES WE EXPERIENCE IN THE LUTEAL PHASE AND THEIR FUNCTION

- Easily startled, hypersensitive to sounds, smells, and social transgressions: More responsive to threats
- Lower energy and motivation to get sh*t done: Conserving energy to fuel pregnancy preparations
- Social withdrawal: Energy conservation, avoidance of communicable illness
- Preferential attention to potential threats: Noticing threats sooner
- Greater tendency to interpret ambiguous events as threats: Reducing the probability of missing threats

tation of this wisdom, helping ensure that we are safe, supported, and have the physical and social resources we need during pregnancy. It is part of our evolutionary success story. And if it's something that we acknowledge and nurture, we can make these changes feel a lot more pleasant than they do for many of us now.

Luteal-Phase Dysregulation and Dysfunction: Why Our PMS Is Worse Than It Was for Our Ancestors

While ignoring our body's changing needs in the luteal phase can create unintentional suffering, this does not mean that we should feel completely terrible. So if you do feel awful in the luteal phase, it may be a sign of dysregulation or disorder. Dysregulation is when PMS is worse than it needs to be because of not-so-amazing environmental changes that have made us less resilient to our hormonal changes than our ancestors were. Disorder is what you get when dysregulation becomes so severe that it turns into PMDD. (PMDD requires special care, and we will discuss it in chapter 10.)

Let's talk about some of the recent environmental changes that have made our cycles worse than they were for our great-great-great-great-grandmothers. Research finds that there are two big classes of environmental change at play. The first stems from the unrealistic expectations of perfection that contemporary society demands of women. The other stems from lifestyle changes that many of us have adopted as we have transitioned from hunter-gatherers to farmers to fast-food consumers and couch-sitters.

First, let's talk about the unrealistic expectation we all have for ourselves to be perfect. This is a pressure that most of us are familiar with. Most of us have been taught from a young age that our value is tied up in our ability to achieve things, and this is true even for those of us whose parents aren't a**holes. We feel that we have to be perfect to be loved and worthy of having good things happen to us. And because we're women, we feel like we have to do all these perfection-creating things while also looking beautiful, put together, and not taking time away from our families to make it all happen. So when we experience a luteal-phase motivational shift*—when it can feel harder to meet the already impossible standards of perfection we set for ourselves—it can seem catastrophic. And when you couple that with the fact that our luteal-phase threat detectors are highly vigilant at this time, it can make us feel as if everything is hopeless. We become angry and frustrated with ourselves for not being productivity robots. And then we become terrified that our failed perfection will make everything we love vaporize into the ether.

As you might expect, all this pressure and self-flagellation makes our luteal-phase mood changes significantly worse than they would be if we didn't have stress-filled, overscheduled lives. Research finds that perfectionism makes cycle-related mood changes worse than they would be in the absence of this drive. And when you add in stress and pressure from work and from family life—which are also related to worsening mood over the course of the luteal phase—it's no wonder we all feel so awful.

Thankfully, the doomsday narratives we tell ourselves, about how we're going to lose everything if we need to slow down a bit from time to time, are nothing more than stories created by our

---

* Note that I am *not* implying that women are impaired in the luteal phase or that we're less able to get things done. It just feels harder when we're doing it.

progesterone-fueled, fear-sensitized brain. Research finds that most women's work-based productivity—except in extreme cases—is not negatively impacted by the hormonal changes across the cycle. The probability that our worlds are going to fall apart because we experience cyclical motivational dips is exceedingly low. Everything that matters to you—your job, your relationships, your family—is not going to vanish into thin air if you ease off the gas pedal a little.* Understanding this and trusting this can create meaningful changes in how we feel during the luteal phase. If we can give ourselves permission to simply acknowledge our feelings for what they are (luteal phase motivational and mood shifts) without needing to punish or hate ourselves, research suggests that we can feel a whole lot better than most of us do now.

The second big change that we have experienced in the last one hundred years or so is that our environments have changed. And these changes have made our brains less able to adapt to our rapidly changing sex hormones than they used to be. Our lack of physical activity, lack of sunlight, heavy reliance on convenience foods, depleted microbiomes, and exposure to chronic stress has created inflammation, decreased neuroplasticity, and left us less able to gracefully navigate the huge hormonal changes that occur in the luteal phase than our ancestors were.

Lacking the ability to quickly adapt to the rising and falling hormone and ALLO levels that characterize the luteal phase can create an experience in our cells that feels like being overwhelmed (when

---

* And not in a lady-of-leisure, I-don't-have-real-responsibilities kind of way. Most of us don't have the luxury of napping in the middle of the day in the luteal phase or being able to delay work deadlines so we can tackle them at a time in the cycle that is more amenable to pulling an all-nighter. There is a middle ground though. The fact is—even on tough work deadline days—we can get a lot more accomplished if we meet ourselves where we are. For me, this usually means taking a deep breath, acknowledging my lower energy level, and slowly but surely putting one foot in front of the other. I get far more accomplished than I do when I am wasting my energy beating myself up for not being on my A game or worrying that I will never be productive again.

there is a lot of hormone/ALLO because it is rising) or being understimulated (when there is not a lot of hormone/ALLO because it is falling). This can make us feel out of sorts and overly sensitive to *everything* as our bodies scramble to adjust. It is what people mean when they talk about progesterone withdrawal being the culprit behind many of the unpleasant premenstrual mood changes that occur right before we start our periods. When we lack resilience to rapid hormonal changes, we can really feel the sudden decrease in progesterone and ALLO. So one way that we can greatly improve the quality of our luteal-phase mood changes is by taking steps to reclaim hormonal flexibility by improving our overall health.

We'll talk more about ways to promote resilience in the face of hormonal change in chapter 11 (feel free to read ahead if anticipating the punchline is distracting), but the message is ultimately as simple as doing things to improve your body's health. This is something we can do without buying any magic potions or having to take up permanent residence at the gym. Research finds that the pillars of cellular plasticity and resilience to hormonal change are as simple as eating food that nourishes our bodies (eating whole, unprocessed foods, with an emphasis on plants), staying physically active, managing our stress, nurturing our relationships, and getting enough sleep and sunlight. It really is that simple (although in our current environment and our contemporary lifestyle, it might not always be easy).

Things You Can Do Today to Start Smoothing Turbulence in Your Luteal Phase

There are a number of things we can do to make our luteal-phase psychological changes feel more like a whisper than a shout. And a lot of them are things that you can start doing today.

- **Track your mood.** Start tracking your mood-related changes across the cycle to learn your unique pattern. I cannot emphasize this enough. Research routinely finds that women differ in the impact hormonal changes across the cycle have on their moods (and this is true for pretty much everything affected by hormones, so brace yourself for the refrain). You can use the cycle-tracking resources I provide in appendix A to start learning your own hormonal rhythms. Alternatively, you can track your mood changes across the cycle (as well as other changes, like changes in libido) using an app like 28. Regardless of how you choose to do it, learning about your hormonal rhythms is the first step toward feeling better across the cycle.

- **Determine whether the emotional changes you experience in the luteal phase are a defense, a dysregulated defense, or a dysfunction.** I define these below:
  - *Defense:* These are the emotional changes you are supposed to feel in the luteal phase, which emerge from our bodies' changing needs and vulnerabilities when pregnant or preparing for pregnancy. This is all that "inherited wisdom from our ancestors" stuff and includes the changes in our energy levels and motivation, as well our increased sensitivity to threats that would be particularly risky in the context of pregnancy (for example, social threats or threats to our security). If you experience an uptick in anxiety and a downshift in mood and motivation, but it is not causing you to stress, then it is normal and part of an evolved defense system to protect us when we're vulnerable and resources are depleted.
  - *Dysregulated defense:* This is where our to-be-expected emotional changes in the luteal phase are turbocharged by environmental changes that make this phase more miserable than what it was for our ancestors. If your luteal phase is frequently characterized by sadness, anger, frustration, anxiety, and feeling unable to cope, and it is causing you problems, it is likely that making some lifestyle

changes might improve how you feel at this time. This is particularly true if you know that there are elements of your diet and lifestyle that might be impairing your body's resilience to hormonal changes (covered in the third bullet point and also in chapter 11).
- *Dysfunction:* If your luteal phase is regularly characterized by crushing sadness, your mood changes across the cycle are interfering with your ability to live your life the way you want to live it, or you find yourself considering self-harm in the luteal phase, you may have PMDD. See chapter 10 to help identify whether this describes you.

- **Take an audit of the things in your life that may be reducing your resilience to hormonal changes.** We will talk more about the specifics of what it looks like to support your hormones with lifestyle choices in chapter 11, but for now, here is a quick list of some of the things that can increase and decrease cellular plasticity and resilience to hormonal changes. Take some time to look at your habits and start by simply taking an audit of what is helping and what is making things worse. And if you're feeling ready, ask yourself: What is one change I can make—that I am willing to make—that will help support my resilience to hormonal changes? Then make that change.

Here are some things to consider adding and subtracting to your life to boost your resilience to hormonal change:
- *Things to add into your life to promote resilience to hormonal change:* meditation, yoga, joy, social support, exercise, getting adequate sleep, eating health-promoting foods (whole, unprocessed, nutrient-dense foods), getting morning sunlight, maintaining a healthy body weight, maintaining insulin sensitivity, stress management, and anything else that decreases inflammation.

- *Things to subtract from your life to promote resilience to hormonal change:* chronic stress, loneliness, processed foods, lack of physical activity, lack of sleep, lack of direct sunlight, lack of nutrients, excess body fat, insulin resistance, and anything else that increases inflammation.

- **Move your body.** If I could give you only one recommendation to make your luteal phase easier to navigate, this would be it. If you are not someone who is physically active, consider starting today. Even taking a walk for thirty minutes most days can be life-changing in terms of improving your mood and building your resilience to hormonal changes. If you aren't able to walk for thirty minutes, start small and build up to that. Walk as far as you can today and every couple of days see if you can add a little more distance. Research finds that exercise is a huge game changer in women's ability to gracefully navigate the hormonal changes across the cycle. If that's not enough to get you sold on exercise, you should also know that research finds that the mood-boosting powers of physical activity are as effective as antidepressants (and without all the terrible side effects). And if you add some strength training in after your walk (especially in the follicular phase, which we will get to in chapter 8), you will help boost testosterone, which is also known for lowering anxiety and increasing well-being.

- **Investigate supplements or dietary changes known to ease cycle-related mood changes.** Although I am not generally a big supplement person (in theory, eating a whole-food, hormone-supporting diet should be sufficient for getting the nutrients we need to be resilient to hormonal changes), there is research that finds certain supplements can improve mood across the cycle. Sometimes extra support is necessary because changes in farming and food-handling practices in the last century have made some nutrients harder to come by than they were for our ancestors. For example, we take in fewer minerals and probiotics from the soil than our ancestors did. (Washing our food washes away bad stuff, but also washes away minerals and good bacteria that our bodies need.) This means that even those of us with the healthiest diets ever can sometimes use additional support. Below are some of the nutrients/herbs that research finds to be supportive of women's moods across the cycle:

- *Chasteberry* (Vitex agnus-castus): This is an herb that has been used for centuries to help women with reproductive-health-related issues. And for good reason: It seems to really work. There are a lot of double-blind, placebo-controlled research studies (the gold standard in clinical research) supporting its effectiveness in managing symptoms of PMS. Typical dosages range from 20 to 40 milligrams of standardized extract (containing 0.5% agnuside) taken once daily. Note that research finds that it can take time for *Vitex* to exert its effects, so it may be several weeks before you notice any improvement. Also note that this is one that you can't get from a food source, so it's Supplement City for you if you'd like to incorporate chasteberry into your life.
- *Magnesium*: This one has more mixed research support (some experiments find that it improves mood in the luteal phase, but others do not). I have included it in this list because it has made a huge difference in my life despite the fact that my diet should not leave me deficient.* It has smoothed out

---

* Research finds that about half of people are deficient. It has been hypothesized that these deficiencies may pop up in people who eat healthy diets because magnesium is abundant in soil, which is something that our ancestors ate a whole lot more of than we do now. So although our changes in food-handling practices have been

the bumps in my luteal-phase mood changes and has also improved the quality of my sleep. So, it works for me. However, given the mixed research support, it may not work for everyone. Some of the most commonly used types of magnesium for smoothing out mood are magnesium glycinate and magnesium citrate. You can also buy broad-spectrum supplements that include multiple types of magnesium (this is what I use; you can learn more about it in appendix C). And if you want to increase your magnesium intake but would rather skip the vitamin aisle, foods rich in magnesium are seeds of all sort (pumpkin, chia), almonds, cashews, spinach, black beans, all things soy, brown rice, avocado, and salmon.*

- *Fish oil or some other omega-3 supplement*: Although you should not need to take an omega-3 supplement if you are eating a diet rich in omega-3 fatty acids (which you can find in things like walnuts, flaxseeds, chia seeds, avocados, and fatty fish like salmon, mackerel, and sardines), there is solid research support that finds that supplementing with omega-3s can improve unpleasant mood changes across the cycle. These improvements also tend to take a little time (a couple of months), so be patient. A recent meta-analysis (which is a study of all the existing studies on a topic) found positive effects of omega-3 supplements on luteal-phase mood using dosages that ranged from 500 to 2,000 milligrams a day, with the most frequently used dose being 2,000 milligrams a day.

---

largely beneficial, it may mean that some of us need to supplement sometimes.
* Writing this made me hungry.

- *Calcium*: Women who experience severe PMS are more likely to have calcium deficiencies than women who do not have PMS. There is also a decent amount of research support suggesting that supplementing with calcium can improve mood in the luteal phase (although a lot of the studies are far from perfect). The typical dosage used in the studies that find positive effects of supplementation were 500 milligrams twice a day. And for those of you looking to increase your calcium intake without a supplement, nondairy[*] sources of calcium are kale (greens of all sort, really), broccoli, sardines, oranges, sesame seeds, white beans, and firm tofu.
- *Vitamin B_6*: Vitamin B_6 is another vitamin that research finds can improve women's moods in the luteal phase. But, as is the case with calcium, we need more research and better-designed studies to draw firm conclusions about its effectiveness as a tamer of hormonal moodiness. The existing evidence, however, supports the idea that it may play a role in improving women's mental health in the luteal phase. The typical dose used in studies finding positive effects on mood is 100 milligrams a day. And if you want to get more B_6 from your food, here are

---

[*] I specify nondairy because most people already know that dairy foods are good sources of calcium, and because I don't like dairy. The reason I don't like it is because (a) some of the proteins in milk like A1 casein are inflammatory and known for causing period problems, (b) milk has hormones like insulin-like growth factor-1 (IGF-1) and prostaglandins that can mess up the functioning of our own endocrine system, and (c) eliminating dairy is often hugely beneficial to women looking to improve their resilience to hormonal changes. So, yeah: I don't like dairy. I don't include it in my diet. And while you are free to make whatever choices feel best for you, I would encourage you to experiment with adding nondairy sources of calcium into your diet as well.

some things known for being boosters of B_6: pork, peanuts, soy-based foods (tofu and edamame), oats, bananas, wheat germ, chickpeas, and dark leafy greens.

If you are going to supplement, try one at a time and see how it makes you feel. Wait a few months before adding the next thing. If you try multiple supplements at the same time, you won't know what's working and what isn't.

- **Be kind to yourself.** If you are feeling a little lower energy or more anxious than you would like in the luteal phase, acknowledge that how you feel is real and recognize that it is temporary. I have found that understanding my feelings as a reflection of the deep evolutionary wisdom of my body trying to manage changing energy needs and vulnerabilities makes them much more tolerable.

- **If you have a romantic partner, communicate.** Research finds that women's luteal-phase experiences improve significantly when they openly acknowledge them to their partners and both partners treat them as normal psychological change. When our partners understand what is happening and why it occurs, it can create a space where we feel like we have permission to use our emotional regulation strategies (e.g., lying down, going for a walk) when we're struggling emotionally. It also eases relationship strain created by emotional turbulence in the luteal phase, which is known to make our mood-related changes feel worse.

  I can't tell you how true this has been for me. Knowing and being able to communicate with my partner that there are seven to ten days each cycle when my danger radar is up has been a 100 percent game changer for me. Having this information doesn't always save me from feeling emotionally turbulent in the luteal phase (I will be the first to admit that, despite having mountains of knowledge about cycles and mood, I am still more likely to lose my sh*t the last two weeks of my cycle than the first), but it always creates a better aftermath. I am quicker to have a follow-up conversation in which I can articulate what set me off and why it made me react the way it did. I can then begin a more productive conversation about the deeper concern that was triggered by my brain's super-sensitive threat detector.

To give you an example of this, my partner and I recently had a blowup over a scheduling error that made me feel like he didn't value time with me. And my luteal-phase brain perceived this as a sign of relationship danger: *Maybe I don't matter very much to him. . . . Am I safe???* So my brain began sounding the danger sirens, and rather than talking through the scheduling error, I blew up. I stormed off to work feeling angry and hurt.

Once I cooled down, I was able to reflect on my reaction. I made note of the fact that I was in the late luteal phase and spent some time thinking about what had happened. I asked myself why his scheduling error set me off (it made me feel unvalued), whether his explanation for the error made sense (it did), and whether the other existing evidence from the course of our relationship supported the view that I am not valued (it did not).

Sometimes, this is all that needs to happen to make me feel better. I can apologize and we can move on with our lives. This time, despite the fact that all the data were adding up to suggest that my fears were not substantiated, my luteal-phase brain still felt threatened. I needed to talk to him and get some extra assurances to calm down my brain. I told him my brain was sounding emergency alarm bells, so I was going to need some extra convincing from him to let me know that I matter and that he values our time together as much as I do.

And you know what? That's exactly what he did. My alarm bells stopped sounding, my amygdala stopped screaming "emergency," and I was able to relax. I addressed the real issue (that my danger centers were reacting to feeling unvalued), which brought me back to a better place. Knowing what was happening internally allowed me to manage the blowup in a productive way. I was able to sincerely apologize to my partner but also be kind to myself about what had happened.

Having both of us attuned to what's going on with my cycle and mood has changed the way we interact on my pricklier days. It hasn't given me license to act like a terrible person (and I'd like to think that I don't). It has just given us an added layer of nuance in our understanding of each other's emotional responses to things.

Although most of us have been taught that our hormonal changes are something to be ashamed of and not discussed in mixed company, this advice is outdated, sexist, and assumes that the male standard for normal should be adopted by all. Being open and communicative about our changing needs across the cycle can minimize conflict and deepen our relationships. It also has the ability to revolutionize the way we address sex and intimacy, which we will turn to next.

CHAPTER 7

SEX AND ATTRACTION ON PROGESTERONE

The great disordering of the female sexual response

At this point in our time together, you should feel pretty well versed in all the fun, flirty things that estrogen does to make us the most sextacular version of ourselves possible in the fertile window. Estrogen makes us look, act, move, sound, and smell sexier to men.* It also makes us more inclined to buy sexier clothes and wear red, and it increases interest in all things sex, flirtation, and sensation seeking than we are when estrogen is low.

Unfortunately, what comes up, must come down. And the flip side of our monthly estrogen-fueled sexiness peak is that most of feel *less* sexually arousable, less sexy, and less turn-on-able at times in the cycle when estrogen levels fall and conception is no longer possible. Research suggests that there is no time in our cycle for which this is more true than the luteal phase. As we transition into the luteal phase our sexual desire hits its cyclical nadir, making us less interested in all things sex and sexiness than we are at other points in our cycle.

For example, in one recent study, researchers followed ninety-seven women and measured their hormone levels, as well as their sexual desire and behavior, every other day for the course of an entire cycle.

---

* This is something that has only been studied in heterosexual men, but I am guessing that lesbian women find their partners sexier at high fertility too.

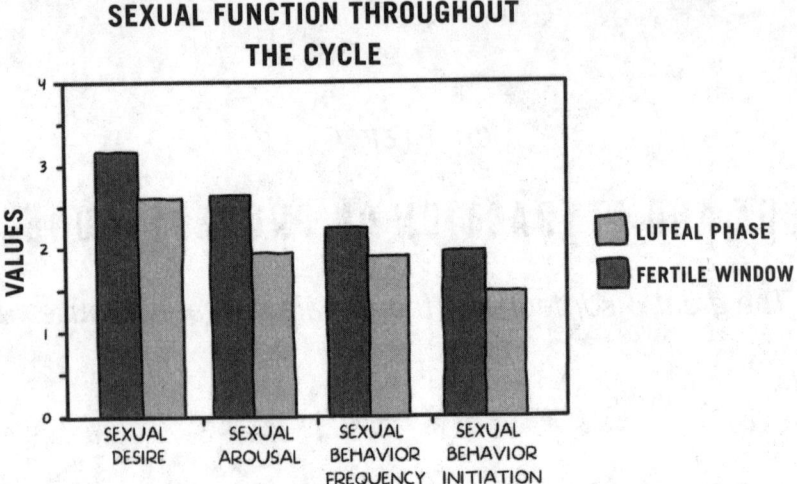

As you can see from the results above, the women reported desiring less sex, having less sex, initiating less sex, and feeling less sexually aroused in the progesterone-fueled luteal phase (light bars) than they did in the estrogen-fueled follicular phase (dark bars).

This general pattern is something that has been observed in dozens of studies now. Women are less sexually interested in the luteal phase than the follicular, making it a relatively nonsexy time in the cycle. These changes are coordinated by a sharp rise in progesterone, which creates changes in the body that are downright sexually antagonistic. For example, it changes the texture of our cervical mucus into something that is thicker, pastier, and less good for sex than the clear, slippery mucus we have in the fertile window. It alters neurotransmission in ways that makes sex less want-able and sexual pleasure less pleasurable. And it also inhibits the activities of 5-alpha-reductase, which is an enzyme that converts testosterone into one of its most potent forms (dihydrotestosterone, aka DHT), which can cut the legs out from under sexual desire, sexual pleasure, and even the frequency and intensity of orgasms.

[Cue the slide whistle here.]

When you've only heard one narrative about what sexual desire is supposed to look like—and it's the one built around the male standard of nonstop turn-on-ability—having a cyclically sensitive sexuality like women have can make us feel like our body isn't doing what it is supposed to. But, for most of us, there isn't something wrong. The release of progesterone cues the beginning of a cycle phase in which (a) sex can no longer lead to conception, and (b) our body is on pregnancy watch. Our decrease in sexual desire and all that goes with it (thicker cervical mucus, etc.) happens as a result of our body shifting its energy away from all things sex and sexiness so that we can direct our energy and attention to preparing for the possibility of pregnancy. And this is what is *supposed* to happen. There is nothing wrong with you, your partner, or your relationship if your sexual desire blinks on and off across the cycle. It is just a manifestation of your brilliant female brain shifting its investment priorities in response to your cycling hormones.

Unfortunately, our decreased investment in all things sex and attraction can feel a little like someone letting the air out of a balloon. Like, here we are, feeling all cute and flirty and then . . . [insert sound of air coming out of a balloon here] . . . it's gone. And the result is that women commonly report feeling less sexy, less desirable, and becoming more critical of themselves in the luteal phase compared to the follicular.

In one study, researchers had women come into the research lab twice: once during the estrogenic fertile window and once again during the luteal phase. At each session, the women were asked questions about their bodies (how desirable they felt and what their most and least favorite body parts were). They also used an eye tracker to measure women's eye movements when looking at themselves in a full-length mirror for three minutes.

Consistent with other research that has come before it, they found that the women reported feeling less desirable in the luteal phase than they did in the follicular. This is the whole air out of the balloon feeling, with women's self-perceptions changing in ways that reflect their bodies' energy shifting away from sex to pregnancy.

They also found that cycle phase influenced what women looked at while gazing at themselves in a mirror. Although women in the fertile window avoided looking at their most disliked body parts, this is *precisely* where women's eyes landed when they were in the luteal phase. Their eyes made a beeline to the parts of their body they reported liking the least and then stayed there. It was like seeing a car crash and not being able to look away. Women who didn't like their hips looked at their hips, women who didn't like their stomach looked at their stomach, and so on. It's almost like they wanted to feel bad about themselves.

Having the sexiness red carpet yanked out from under our feet when estrogen crashes can be pretty jarring and make us feel not great about our physical appearance. And when the ego-boosting powers of estrogen get replaced by the negatively charged, alarm-bell-ringing powers of progesterone, it can make us more worried about and critical of our imperfections. We are more likely to fixate on the parts we wish we could improve and are less willing to appreciate the things that make us beautiful.

If you feel less sexy and more critical of yourself during the last two weeks of your cycle, it's not just you. It's most of us. I can't tell you the number of women who tell me they feel "gross," "disgusting," or as one woman put it, "completely unf*ckable"* in the luteal phase. Women's sexual desire usually has more to do with how they feel about *themselves* than it does with how they feel about their partners. So when we feel gross, disgusting, or unsexy, it can send our already sleepy luteal-phase libido into complete sexual lockdown.

Of Mice and (Wo)men

I wouldn't need to dedicate an entire chapter to sexual desire in the luteal phase if the entirety of the story was *women-don't-want-to-have-sex-as-much-in-the-luteal-phase-and-that's-it-okay-bye*. While there is little doubt that women are less sexually turn-on-able in the luteal phase than the follicular, the surprising thing is that human females have a

---

* Don't shoot the messenger.

lot more luteal-phase sex than most of our closest primate relatives do. Our closest primate relatives—like gorillas, geladas, baboons, and macaques—limit most of their sexual activity to the fertile window (plus or minus a few days for good measure). They do this because it's too costly to be a pastime of choice when it won't lead to conception. The fact that human females continue to be as sexually motivated as most of us are in the luteal phase is something that makes us different from most of the other mammals in the world.

So, what's up with all the sex that human females have in the luteal phase?

The answer to this riddle turned up in (of all places) the brain of a cute little rodent called the prairie vole (aka *Microtus ochrogaster*), which lives in grasslands in the midwestern US. Prairie voles have gotten a lot of research play from evolutionary biologists and neuroscientists because they have more than a few things in common with humans. They tend to form long-term, mostly monogamous relationships. Their relationships are characterized by shared living space, joint rearing of offspring, and mutual investment in the other's well-being. And, like humans, bonds between partners are typically exclusive, with mated pairs showing a strong preference for their partner over alternative mates. They're kind of like the 1940s television sitcom family of the rodent world.

Another thing that makes prairie voles like humans is that they have sex across the cycle. They have sex during the females' fertile window (like all sexually reproducing species do), but they also have sex outside of it (which most sexually reproducing species do not). And it is from the study of prairie voles that researchers have been able to break down the evolutionary wisdom of luteal-phase sexual activity and learn about the nonreproductive functions of sex.

Although there are a number of functions that sex can serve in a relationship, evolutionarily the primary benefit that sex seems to provide couples is that it keeps them together. From the study of voles, we have learned that the neural pathways linked to sexual arousal and sexual satisfaction also serve as the building blocks of lasting relationship satisfaction. The sexual release of neurotransmitters and hormones like oxytocin and vasopressin—which we release when we have sex—don't just reinforce sexual behavior, they also promote attachment to our partners. Sex, in addition to reproduction, helps to promote attachment, partnership, and commitment, all of which are necessary for the shared care of offspring.

Luteal-phase sex is about strengthening the relationship bond, and having bonded relationships is something that humans are favored to do because of the absolutely unbridled neediness of our babies. They are among the neediest and most dependent in the entire animal kingdom. In fact, their extreme neediness is believed to be the evolutionary raison d'être behind humans' evolving to form pair-bonds in the first place. Historically, there was just no way that any one human being could possibly meet all of a tiny human's needs on their own.* One of the ways that women were able to improve the survival chances of their children—as well as their continued success as adults—was to form long-term, stable pair-bonds with partners who were able to help share the demands of provisioning and childcare. And sex is an important part of this picture. Several decades of research has now verified the fact that, for humans, sex plays an important role in creating and helping maintain happy, lasting relationships.

In one study, researchers tested whether the warm-fuzzy love haze we get from sex—sexual afterglow—helps cement couples together by increasing relationship satisfaction, even after the sex is finished and our clothes are on. To study this, they had 214 newlywed couples keep diaries for fourteen days. Each day, they reported whether they had sex and how satisfied they were with their sex life. The couples also reported on their global relationship satisfaction at the beginning and end of the fourteen days and then again four to six months later.

They found that in most couples, sex on a given day predicted in-

---

* If you have a child/children, you know this to be totally true. There are literally not enough hours in the day for any one person to do all the caregiving required for young children. It's brutal. And for our female ancestors, who didn't have access to the same sorts of resources we do now (we can order food and hire childcare), it would have been even harder.

creased relationship satisfaction that extended for two full days after sex had occurred (i.e., a sexual afterglow). More importantly, they found that although it was typical for the couples to experience a slight decline in relationship satisfaction over time (this happens in newlywed couples when the relationship begins to lose its new-car smell), the strength of their reported postsex afterglow served as a buffer against a steep decline. Couples with the strongest sexual afterglow had the highest relationship satisfaction at the end of the study. Sex, and the lingering feeling of satisfaction we continue to get from sex, helps to solidify bonds and promote bonding. So although biologists tend to focus on sex being all about reproduction and getting genes passed down from one generation to the next, it also serves the important function of creating connection.

This, my friends, is the zone of genius for the luteal phase.

Although women receive bonding-related benefits from sex regardless of where they are in their cycles, sex in the luteal phase is *all* about bonding and relationship building. That's the primary function it serves. So, while it is clear that women in the estrogenic fertile window are more sexually motivated than women in the luteal phase, progesterone doesn't completely obliterate sexual desire altogether. It just changes the nature of our sexual motivations. It decreases that sort of *I-need-an-orgasm-right-now-and-better-you-than-my-vibrator* spontaneous sexual desire that tends to characterize the fertile window, replacing it with sexual desire that is motivated by the need for connection. And research finds when women are in the luteal phase, one of the big motivational forces that drives their initiated sexual behavior is the need to connect and feel close to their partners.

For example, in one study, researchers followed fifty heterosexual couples and looked at changes in sexual desire over the cycle based on the degree to which each member of the pair was invested in the relationship. The latter was measured by asking each member of the couple about the extent to which they felt invested in their partner and the extent to which they felt their partner was invested in them. They then measured the couples' self-reports of sexual behavior—and who initiated the sexual behavior—over the course of a cycle.

Given that the luteal phase is regularly found to be linked with lower sexual desire and less sexual behavior than what is found in the follicular, they predicted that, on the whole, this would be the pattern they'd observe in their sample. However, given that luteal-phase sex can be used as a tool for creating intimacy and fostering relationship investment, they predicted that the magnitude of this decrease would be influenced in important ways by women's relationship-investment needs. Specifically, rather than seeing all women experience a luteal-phase decrease in sexual desire, they predicted that those women who felt the biggest need to create connection with their partners (i.e., women who felt that their partners were less invested in their relationships than they were themselves) would continue to experience relatively high sexual desire and continue to initiate sex with their partners at a high rate once they moved from the follicular phase into the luteal phase.

And this is exactly what they found. Although, on the whole, women's sexual behavior decreased as they entered into the luteal phase from the fertile window, the decrease wasn't something experienced equally across all women in the study. Women who felt that their partners were less invested in their relationships than they were themselves—whose need to cement the relationship was greatest—continued to maintain high levels of sexual desire across the cycle. They also continued to seek sex with their partners out of the fertile window to a much greater extent than women who felt they were more equally invested in the relationship. For these women, the need for luteal-phase sex was less necessary, since the need to cement the bond was lower. Sex is a good way for those of us in need of connection to unleash some vasopressin and oxytocin within ourselves and our partners to help strengthen the connection and bond we have in our relationships. And there is no time in which we are more inclined to have this sort of need than in the luteal phase. During this phase, women are more prone to anxiety about their relationships (remember from the last chapter?), and this is one of the ways they can soothe their anxiety and quiet the alarm bells.

These shifts occur because progesterone shifts the body into pregnancy-preparation mode. In the same way that it causes the cells in the endometrium to change in ways that create the most hospitable environment inside for a pregnancy, progesterone also causes the cells in the brain to work together to orient our brains and behaviors toward creating a hospitable environment outside for pregnancy (and childcare). Sex with our partners—because it helps solidify our relationships and ensure their continued investment in us and our existing or assumed future offspring—is part of this picture. Because of this, sex can feel particularly comforting and rewarding to the luteal-phase brain.

AN INTERESTING THING ABOUT ORGASMS (YOU KNOW, SINCE WE'RE HERE)

Although all of us have been taught that orgasms are the quintessential pot of gold at the end of the sexual rainbow, research suggests women's brains might not see it that way. Although orgasms are the thing that motivates men's brains to seek out sex, this isn't true for women. For us, it's the other stuff—the *reasons* that we're having sex (whether it's to experience pleasure, feel connected to our partners, or something else altogether)—that is pivotal in motivating our wanting of sex and the degree to which our brain finds it rewarding. If we're having sex to connect and it makes us feel connected, our brains feel rewarded and we'll want to do it again in the future. No orgasm required. The cultural messaging that equates having an orgasm with good sex and not having an orgasm with bad sex doesn't fit for women. It just puts unnecessary pressure on women to have nonstop orgasms, which isn't something that all women's bodies are equipped to do. Research finds that around 50–70 percent of women do not consistently achieve orgasm through intercourse alone, and 10–40 percent of women rarely have them at all. Sex isn't always about reproduction (thank you, prairie voles, for that important lesson), and really good sex isn't always about orgasms.

Luteal-phase sex and sexual desire are driven by a categorically different type of unconscious psychological calculus than estrogenic fertile-window sex and sexual desire. It's motivated by different needs (the need to connect versus the need for pleasure, excitement, and a sexy adventure). And it's more likely to be highly partner-specific. Although the estrogenic sexual desire tends to be targeted toward our partner as well as whoever happens to be the hottest guy in the room (estrogen is known to make our eyes wander . . . and although we don't usually act on that, the wandering is real), progesterone is all about *your* partner. It's about connection. It's about strengthening the bond. And it's about creating the type of relationship with a partner that will provide a nurturing environment for pregnancy and raising children.

I Lust You, I Lust You Not

Progesterone affects our sexual desire and sexual motivation in ways that reflect the shifting costs and benefits of sex in the luteal phase, but this isn't where the impact of progesterone's effects on our sexual and relationship psychology ends. Because in addition to making us feel like a less-sexy, less-easily arousable version of ourselves, it also changes the types of qualities that we are most drawn to in men. Research suggests that our two hormones work together in the context of partner choice, with each specializing in sharpening our brain's attunement to the qualities that pack the biggest punch in terms of promoting successful conception (estrogen) and pregnancy/childcare (progesterone).

In the estrogenic follicular phase, sex is about getting the best genes possible for our children. This isn't what's usually going on consciously, of course (at least not most of the time[*]), but we have

---

[*] Although some of the time, this is exactly what is going on consciously in women's brains: "That man would give me beautiful children" is something I have heard come out of more than one woman's mouth.

inherited partner preferences that zero in on qualities related to good genes in the fertile window because that is when conception is possible, and if there is ever a time that it pays for us to focus on good genes, this is it. Over the course of our evolutionary history, those women who just so happen to be drawn to men with the best-quality genes at times in the cycle when conception was possible would have passed down a greater number of genes than those whose preferences were more "gene neutral." This is because the good genes–focused women, on average, would have had healthier children than those belonging to the gene-neutral women. Over time, the preference for good-gene qualities at high fertility is something that would have been handed down over and over again because all those women who inherited this tendency would be healthy enough to have children of their own.

So, what sorts of traits speak to the quality of a potential partner's genes? One possible marker of this is testosterone. The reason testosterone cues speak to genetic quality is because it is traded off with immune function (meaning that when one goes up, the other goes down). This means that only men with particularly efficient immune genes can afford to release a lot of it. Women find qualities like chiseled jaws and broad shoulders sexy, in part because the men who have these qualities are advertising that their immune genes are so bada*s and high functioning that they were able to release copious amounts of testosterone throughout development without any issue. Our heads turn at the sight of men who have these qualities—particularly when we are in the fertile window, because our brain is trying to get us to choose partners with good genes for our children at times when conception is possible. And several lines of research have found evidence that our preference for these types of qualities in men[*] experiences a significant uptick when estrogen is rising and conception is possible.

---

[*] For heterosexual women. Unfortunately, we don't yet know much about this in lesbian women. Interestingly (and this is anecdotal, so take it with a grain of salt), I have bisexual friends who note that their interest in men goes up near the fertile window and is at its lowest in the luteal phase.

The luteal phase is a little different, however. While sex in the estrogenic follicular phase is all about sex for the sake of sex and attraction for the sake of good genes, in the luteal phase sex is a reproductive dead-end, and the quality of a person's genes no longer matters. As a result of this, our sexual motivation shifts from being all about signs of genetic quality to being something that strikes a greater balance between our desire for good genes and our desire for a partner who possesses the types of qualities that would make them a good partner and father to our children.

In one study, researchers had women interact with two men (who were actually actors hired by the researchers). One was a somewhat average-looking guy who possessed "good dad" qualities (stability, reliability, expressed an interest in getting married and having children). The other was a sexy, devil-may-care type who exuded confidence, good-gene markers, and made it very clear by the things he said that he had no interest in a long-term relationship (let alone fathering). The women interacted with the men twice, once in the estrogenic fertile window, and once in the progestogenic luteal phase. The researchers recorded the women's interactions with each of the men at each cycle phase and had them scored for flirting behavior.

Women in the fertile window exhibited a clear preference for the sexy good-genes guy relative to his more average-looking "good dad" counterpart. But when progesterone came storming on the scene in the luteal phase, that preference disappeared. Women demonstrated equal amounts of flirtatiousness with each of the two men, with a slight preference for the good dad. Similar patterns are found when looking at women's preferences for men's faces and voices as well. While estrogen puts the pedal to the metal on our preference for testosterone markers, progesterone balances our preferences in ways that deemphasize the desire for good genes and increases our desire for investment potential.

We exhibit these changes because provisioning and investment have played such a huge role in our ancestors' ability to get their genes passed down from one generation to the next. Although the quality of our partners' genes matter, these other qualities have been just as important—if not more so—in the ultimate success of our genetic lineage. This is also why we see that progesterone tends to be associated with our brain's response to monetary rewards. Although progesterone has the general effect of dimming our response to pleasure and decreasing how motivated we are to get pleasurable things (that dopamine-driven "wanting" response that we talked about in chapter 6), research finds that monetary rewards—which are the ultimate contemporary symbol of safety and security—are greater in the late luteal phase compared to what is seen in the follicular. Our brains are all about security, stability, and all the other qualities that help ensure that we will have access to the resources we need to have a successful pregnancy and be able to care for children.

So how does this actually play out in relationships and when choosing partners? Well, I can tell you it does *not* mean that we're flighty or fickle . . . or that we feel the need to switch out partners every fourteen days (Mr. Hottt Sexysex for Days 1–14 and then Mr. Caring Reliable for Days 15–28).* Instead, it simply means that our hormonal changes will help us choose partners who possess both sets of qualities because each cycle phase gets a "vote." Having our preferences nudged back and forth between prioritizing good genes and prioritizing investment allows us to exercise balance in our choice of partners. We will choose partners who hit enough of our good-gene buttons to appease our estrogenic brain. And we will choose someone who hits enough of our investment and commitment buttons to make our luteal-phase brain happy too.

Our shifting sexual psychology can also turn the volume up and down on the types of things that attract us and annoy us about partners we have or those we're pursuing. Although there is very little research on how hormonal changes in attraction play out in the context of long-term relationships, there is every reason to predict that they have some impact on the daily waxing and waning of feelings that go on—and are totally normal—in romantic relationships.

---

* This isn't to say that the thought might not cross our minds from time to time (although if you ever tell anyone I said that, I will deny it every time).

Anything that highlights our partner's testosterone levels is likely to be noticed and appreciated by our estrogenic brain in the fertile window. We may find ourselves feeling suddenly luststruck by our partner when the light hits their jawline just so, we overhear them taking charge on a work call, or we see them doing something else that requires strength or skill. Conversely, if our partners fail to take control of a situation or exhibit some other momentary lapse of leadership that temporarily casts their genetic quality in an unfavorable light . . . well . . . I'm guessing it probably bothers us a whole lot more than it would in the luteal phase, and if it is someone we have just started dating, it may even give us the ick.

In the luteal phase, on the other hand, it's likely that we're more apt to appreciate our partners' provisioning, partnering, and fathering qualities then we are in the follicular. And we are also more likely to be easily upset by any signs suggesting that investment may be lacking. For example, we should feel particularly drawn to and appreciative of our partners when they demonstrate that they love and care for us. And the types of issues that are most likely to cause relationship turbulence are those stemming from a perceived lack of care, investment, and willingness to commit to us and any children we may bear.

Research is just beginning to understand the way that our hormonal changes affect our relationship dynamics and attraction. Keeping track of how your own attraction and sexual psychology change across your cycle can be incredibly effective at helping you navigate your changing feelings across the cycle. Knowing what will pull you in and push you away sexually can help you set up the dynamics in your relationship in ways that promote long-term attraction and relationship satisfaction (if this is what you are going for) or can prevent you from getting hurt if you want to keep things casual (given our luteal-phase needs, there is little doubt that short-term sexual encounters feel less fun in the luteal phase than the follicular). When you know your cycle, you can know yourself. And when we know ourselves, it makes it possible for us to have a lifetime of great sex and meaningful relationships.

Things You Can Do Today to Support Your Luteal-Phase Sexuality

Just like we did with mood, we are going to go over some of the things that you can do today to help support your luteal-phase sexuality, because it can be hard when we don't feel sexy and our sex drive is feeling sort of meh. Here are a few things to get you started in supporting the sexual side of things during the back half of your cycle:

- **Track your sexual desire across the cycle.** If you aren't already tracking your sexual desire across the cycle, I encourage you to start now. Use the cycle-tracking resources I have linked in appendix A or use an app like 28 to guide you. This is important because each of us is a little bit different. Although many women follow the evolutionarily predictable pattern, in which sexual desire increases near ovulation and then falls (sometimes rather spectacularly) in the luteal phase, this isn't true for everyone. For some of us, sexual desire marches to the beat of its own drum . . . and that drum isn't necessarily playing a tune in which sexual desire is highest in the fertile window when estrogen peaks.
- **If you have a partner, communicate.** This is particularly important if you have a male partner because many of them don't have a clue what it's like to have dual sexuality (guided by two hormones instead of one). They can take it personally when our sexual desire seems to blink on and off like a streetlight on a timer because their sexual desire doesn't usually decrease unless there is a problem. Teaching your partner about the ebb and flow of your sexual desire can be a real game changer for men. It can create a space where they no longer perceive your changing sexual needs as emblematic of something they're doing wrong or a problem with the relationship. Instead, it becomes something that the two of you can navigate as a couple.

You may also find it helpful to communicate with your partner about how the meaning of sex can change across the cycle—communicating that you need closeness in the luteal phase more than mind-blowing orgasms can make it easier for you to get what you want out of any sexual encounter. It can also help your partner understand why the idea of sneaking in a quickie on your lunch break without any buildup or after-snuggle probably isn't going to push the right buttons in the luteal phase, even if it was exactly what you needed the week before in the fertile window.

- **Do health and relationship checks.** Sexual desire and sexual function are experiences that are both embodied (meaning that they are created by and experienced by the physical body) and relational (meaning that they emerge in response to another person). One of the best things we can do to support sexual desire across the cycle is to be vigilant about maintaining the health of our bodies and our relationships.

First, do a health check. Our physical bodies, including our brain (remember: it's a body part too!), are responsible for creating the experience of attraction and sexual desire. This means that one of the very best things that we can do to keep our sex lives smoothly humming along across the cycle is to keep our bodies healthy and strong. There is so, *so* much research linking sexual desire and sexual function to physical fitness and health. One of the simplest ways we can support seamless transitions in sexual desire across the cycle is by taking steps to improve the health of our bodies (see chapter 11 for ideas about where to start).

Next, do a relationship audit. If you are struggling with sexual desire, ask yourself whether there are any unresolved issues in your relationship that could be getting in the way. Research generally finds that low sexual desire in women (whether in or out of the luteal phase) stems from unresolved relationship problems interfering with attraction.

And because our threat detector is extra sensitive in the season of progesterone, this is a time when our unresolved issues can feel larger than life, dampening our attraction to our partners and making our sex drive disappear into the vapor. Being vigilant about maintaining the health of our relationships is good for your luteal-phase brain's peace of mind and is also good for sex.

- **Fight the good fight (or don't!) against feeling unsexy.** Unfortunately, it is very common for women to feel unsexy during the luteal phase. This can be really hard. It can make us overly critical of our appearance and make us feel bad about ourselves. Although there is not a ton of research out there about ways we can get out of feeling this way, there is some evidence that self-compassion (talking to yourself with kindness and reminding yourself that your feelings are temporary) and gratitude (writing about or vividly imagining the things we are grateful for) can make us feel better when we're having an "I'm so gross" day.

  For me, I have found that simply reminding myself that how I feel, though real, is a product of my brain and not a product of reality is super helpful in getting me out of a counterproductive "I'm so disgusting" narrative. Acknowledging the reasons why I feel as I do (my perception is distorted by the fact that I've had an estrogen crash and the fear centers of my brain are primed) allows me not to fixate on feeling that way and to move on to other things. I have also found that leaning into my luteal phase, rather than fighting against it, helps me feel more comfortable in my skin when I am feeling icky. I don't try to fight against how I'm feeling by wearing my sexiest dress or my highest heels to see if I can bring sexy back. That usually makes me feel worse. Instead, I'll put on my favorite leggings and sweatshirt and lean into the luteal-phase slowdown.

- **Get outside of yourself by dropping into a fantasy.** It's so, so common for women to feel less sexy in the season of progesterone. And, as noted, this isn't something that a lot of us can talk ourselves out of by wearing our favorite hot-girl outfit or telling ourselves how sexy we are. During these times, know that you don't need to have any sex that you don't feel like having. But for these times when you're feeling about as sexy as your grandmother's couch and *want* to feel sexy, I offer you a workaround to get in the mood: Get outside yourself altogether. Not in a dissociation/defense mechanism sort of way, but in more of a "diving headfirst in a great sexual fantasy" kind of way. The sort of thing that allows you to experience sexual desire as the sexy, sexual-fantasy version of yourself rather than the version of you that is in threadbare sweatpants eating peanut butter straight out of the jar (or maybe that's just me right now).

If you are looking to get things going but don't know where to start, companies like Dipsea and Quinn offer female-forward audio erotica that can help you get the ball rolling. Or, if you like to do things the old-fashioned way, there are always trashy novels, the internet, and your own scandalous imaginings (I know you've got it in you). Thinking about sex in a way that removes you from the center of it all can help fan the flames of desire when we're not feeling sexy enough for sex, which can be common in the luteal phase.

- **Investigate supplements or dietary changes to improve sexual function.** Again, I want to add my caveat that often supplements are not necessary (and eating a nutrient-dense, hormone-supporting diet should have you meeting your nutrient needs); however, there are some supplements that research suggests might help if you are looking for extra support:
  - *Maca root:* Maca root is a plant native to the Peruvian Andes that has been used for almost a thousand years to support sexual functioning and libido. Although

it's only relatively recently that maca's effects on sexual function have begun to be systematically studied, the results look promising. There is research suggesting some beneficial effects on sexual desire and function in both men and women. It's also been found to be helpful in restoring libido in response to the use of antidepressants containing selective serotonin reuptake inhibitors (SSRIs). I wouldn't be a good scientist if I didn't add the caveat that research support for maca isn't 100 percent conclusive. Some studies find positive effects on libido and sexual function while others don't. But I know many women who use it and love it, so it may be worth learning more about if you are looking for additional support for your sexual desire. Typical dosages used in research are 3.5 to 5 grams of maca root powder taken once daily, or 500 to 1,000 milligram capsules taken three times a day. As with most things, it can take a few weeks for you to experience positive effects.

- Tribulus terrestris: *Tribulus terrestris* is a plant that has been used in traditional medicine in China and India for centuries to support sexual health and overall vitality. There is decent research support—including from randomized, placebo-controlled clinical trials (that scientific gold standard)—that it may be helpful for boosting female sexual desire.* Studies on *Tribulus terrestris* have used a wide range of doses, ranging anywhere from 250 milligrams to more than 1,000 milligrams per day, so you should

---

* Although, as a caveat, note that most of the research on this supplement has been conducted on menopausal women. While there is reason to expect that it would have comparable effects on premenopausal women who are having problems with sexual desire, we do not know that for certain.

talk to a health-care professional to get a targeted recommendation if you are interested in trying it. And, as always with supplements, the effects are not going to be immediate, so if you try it, be patient. Results often take several weeks.

- *Vitamin D*: Vitamin D is one of those nutrients in the body that's involved in almost every system we have. So when we are deficient, there is a lot of sh*t that can go sideways in the body, including sexual desire and sexual function. Research finds that women with sexual desire dysfunction are significantly more likely to have vitamin D deficiencies than are women with healthy levels of desire. There is also some (limited) evidence that supplementing with vitamin D may improve women's sexual functioning. One of the first things you can do to support your sexual function is get your vitamin D checked. This is especially true for people of color. Melanin acts as a natural sunscreen and reduces the skin's ability to synthesize vitamin D. This is great for minimizing cellular damage from the sun, but less good for synthesizing vitamin D. If your vitamin D levels are low, take steps to address it. If you are looking to boost your vitamin D naturally, spend more time outside. Our bodies have the ability to synthesize all the vitamin D they need from exposure to sunlight (a lot of us are deficient in this vitamin simply because we don't spend as much time outside as our ancestors did). Having your arms and legs exposed to sunlight for about ten to thirty minutes (less for fair skin, more for dark skin) two to three times per week is about all that you need to meet your body's vitamin D needs. If you want to go the supplement route, a typical daily dose of vitamin D used in supplements ranges from 600 to 2,000 IU

(15 to 50 micrograms). There can be too much of a good thing with vitamin D, so make sure to use caution and talk to your doctor or other health-care professional if you are considering using more than the standard dosage.

Let me close this chapter by saying that it is totally normal, natural, and even functional (remember: sex is germy and metabolically costly!) to experience changing sexual desire across the cycle. Although many of us have been led to believe that there is something wrong with being anything other than 100 percent turn-on-able all the time, this just isn't a pattern that would make any sense at all for a person with a female body.

Our interest in sex, our reasons for wanting sex, how we feel about ourselves, and the qualities that we are most drawn to in our existing or prospective partners changes with our changing hormones. The best sex of our lives will come from embracing the duality of our sexuality and communicating about our changing needs to ensure that we're getting what we need from our relationships on all twenty-eight-ish days of our cycle.

CHAPTER 8

NUTRITION, EXERCISE, SLEEP, AND RECOVERY

Advice for the luteal phase

If you're a woman, I'm guessing you're not exactly a wellspring of self-love and positivity when it comes to your body. This is something that tends to be true for us even if we don't buy into diet culture BS or feel the need to look like whatever ideal is being pushed by our social media feed. Research finds that by the time girls reach their seventeenth birthday, 78 percent report being unhappy with their bodies. And somewhere between 69 and 84 percent of women continue to feel this way as adults. This means that if (a) you're a woman, and (b) you have a body, there's a good chance you've already spent a lot of time wishing yours looked different than it does.

Most of us don't just feel unhappy with how our bodies look. We also feel unhappy with how they feel. We can't understand why we feel so tired and hungry all the time. Or why our bodies don't respond to our gym time with fitness gains that match the magnitude of how miserable we feel when we're slogging through our exercise routine. Sometimes, it seems like the more we try to do things right, the worse we feel. We can't understand why we're hungrier and more tired when we're following all the advice we've been given by experts than we do when we're ignoring them. But rather than questioning the advice we've been given, we instead learn to distrust our bodies' signals. We become conditioned to see our body as the enemy that is standing in the way of good health and fitness.

Almost every woman I know has felt way. *I* have felt this way. Where it feels like the one thing standing between ourselves and our health and wellness goals is our own body. Which doesn't make any sense at all. Not only *are* we our bodies (your brain is a body part, making the body-as-an-enemy paradigm a war with only one side), it feels really confusing to think that our body would be giving us a bum steer when it comes to taking care of itself. I mean, shouldn't our bodies *want* to do the things that will help to keep them healthy?

Now, it is true that sometimes our body will want us to do things that are counterproductive to health. This can happen because our brains and bodies are optimized for surviving and reproducing in environments that are pretty different from our own. This is called an evolutionary mismatch, which is what happens when the speed of changes in the environment outpaces evolutionary change, leading us to respond to things in ways that are bad for us. This is very much the case with our brain when it comes to food. We have a brain that falls immediately in love with all things fatty and sugary because for most of our history eating such things would have helped our bodies get the nutrients we needed to survive. And then if there were any calories in excess, we could store them on our bodies as fat, which would help withstand food shortages during times when resources were scarce.

In our current environment, of course, these tendencies can get us into trouble. This is because much of the food (or "food") in our current environment is full of fat and sugar, which hits our brain's reward buttons without providing much nourishment. We eat and eat but continue to feel hungry because these fake foods lack fiber and don't stretch the mechanoreceptors in our stomach that tell us to stop eating. Additionally, the nutrient-sensing neurons in our gut* will tell

---

* These are called neuropods and this is, in my mind, some of the coolest research being done in neuroscience right now. The work of Dr. Diego Bohórquez and his lab at Duke is particularly fascinating and on the cutting edge of this new field of work.

the brain that we need to keep eating even after our calorie needs are met because our nutrient needs are coming up short.

Some of our frustration with our bodies is the result of the fact that our neural circuits don't recognize processed food to be a nutritional trap. This can get us stuck in a vicious cycle of craving, eating, and self-flagellation that makes us angry with ourselves and certain that our body is the enemy. But for women, there is more to our body frustration than that. There are a lot of us who struggle with feeling tired and hungry even when eating healthy foods and exercising regularly. And this can create frustration and confusion over the fact that our bodies seem to want to lead us in the wrong direction when it comes to our health.

So why do so many of us struggle with low energy and food cravings when we're doing everything right? It's actually very simple. It's because the rules we've been given to follow in the name of good nutrition and fitness—for lack of a more diplomatic way to say it—make no f*cking sense whatsoever for women. They weren't made for our bodies. They were made for men. And because our bodies' needs change across the cycle, one-size-fits-all rules don't work well for us when it comes to exercise and nutrition. They make us hungry, tired, and teach us to distrust our bodies when they're telling us we need something different. Because when we spend half our time still hungry after eating the number of calories we've been told to eat . . . and feel depleted rather than energized after going to the gym . . . it can seem like our body is working against us and can't be trusted.

If you are a female with a cycle, your hormonal changes impact your nutrition and exercise needs. Following nutrition and fitness guidance designed for men is going to set us up for failure, *especially* in the luteal phase. This is because the luteal phase is uniquely female. There is no biological analogue in men. This makes the health and fitness guidelines designed for men (which most of them are) particularly ill-suited for women's bodies during this time. They leave us overworked and underfed, leading to exhaustion and preoccupation with food as our body tries to right the wrongs imposed by wellness guidelines that don't work for us.

Food, Fat, and Fertility

To understand why our nutrition and exercise needs differ so much across the cycle, the first thing we need to talk about is how costly reproduction is for those of us with female bodies. Although this is something that we all know on some level, the extent to which this is true may surprise you. For example, in humans, a nine-month pregnancy generally requires an extra 350–450 calories a day to sustain. And breastfeeding—which was a nonnegotiable for our female ancestors—requires something along the lines of an extra 500–700 calories a day (an investment that is generally required for at least the first year of a child's life, but likely two to three years for our ancestors). There is nothing that any organism will ever do that even comes close to being as metabolically expensive as reproduction for a female mammal.

Interestingly enough, the huge energy costs of reproduction actually start *before* an egg is even fertilized. This is true even if your sex life or partner preferences completely preclude the possibility of pregnancy altogether. If you ovulate and progesterone is released, your body will begin the costly act of turning itself into the sort of respectable establishment that's appropriate for a baby to grow in, whether you have any plans for pregnancy or not. And this is no small job. It requires the growth of new tissue in places like the breasts and endometrium to make them suitable for housing and feeding our young. It also requires making adjustments to everything else our bodies do (things like circulating blood and fighting off germs) to accommodate the fact that we may soon have to share our body with another person, whom we also must construct. These are energy-demanding tasks. As a result, our heart rate, respiration rate, and energy use while resting all increase in the luteal phase compared to the follicular.

For example, in one study, researchers had naturally cycling women come into the research laboratory twice, once in the follicular phase of the cycle and once again in the luteal phase. At each session, wom-

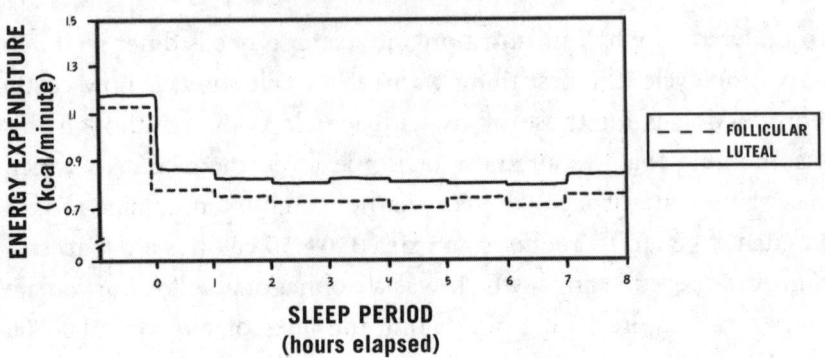

en's body temperature, respiration rate, and resting metabolic rate were continuously measured throughout the night while the women slept. And as you can see from the figure above, they found significant differences in how hard women's bodies were working while they slept that were cycle-phase dependent. When the women were in the luteal phase, their core body temperature was higher, their respiration rate was faster, and (as shown above) they burned a significantly greater number of calories than they did when they were in the follicular phase.

This isn't the only study to observe this pattern. Research regularly finds that women's bodies work harder and can burn up to 11 percent more calories in the luteal phase compared to the follicular. And these are differences that matter. A person with a 2,000-calorie-a-day diet needs an additional 140–175 calories daily to help offset the metabolic cost. Progesterone makes us hardworking, energy-burning machines.

The natural result of this increased energy need is that our bodies are going to want to eat more. Our bodies—when left to their own devices and fed healthy foods—will generally regulate energy homeostatically, which means balancing the energy we burn with the energy we take in. Progesterone increases appetite to help ensure that energy needs are increasing during this time when energy expenditure is high. Which is why research regularly finds that females in species ranging from rats and guinea pigs to great apes and humans feel hungrier and eat more in the luteal phase than they do in the follicular.

For example, in one study, researchers measured two groups of women eating lunch, one group in the luteal phase and the other in the follicular phase, to see whether there was evidence of cycle-based differences in appetite. When they compared the amount of food that was consumed by the two groups of women, they found that the average luteal-phase meal had 172 more calories than what was present in the follicular-phase meals (810 calories in the luteal; 638 in the follicular). This general pattern is something that has been repeated in several studies using multiple types of measures. In one recent review of thirty-seven different published research studies examining the relationship between cycle phase and food intake, researchers found that women ate more in the luteal phase than follicular in all but two of the studies. Similar results are found in nonhuman females, some of whom have pregnancies that are far less costly than ours. One study found that rats eat approximately 20–25 percent more chow during the rat equivalent of the luteal phase* than during their version of the follicular phase, reflecting their body's changing energy needs as they prepare for reproduction.

Mechanistically, these changes are caused by progesterone increasing GABAergic activity in the brain and decreasing insulin sensitivity. When GABA receptors are stimulated, they slow down the brain, and (interestingly enough) slowed-down brains take longer to hit the brakes on hunger when we're eating. So progesterone, through its increased activation of our GABA receptors, makes it so we're slower to get full.

Progesterone also increases appetite by decreasing insulin sensitivity. Insulin is a hormone produced by the pancreas that helps regulate blood-sugar levels. When you eat, carbohydrates are broken down into glucose, which enters the bloodstream. From there, insulin signals cells throughout the body—especially in the liver, muscles, and fat tissue—to absorb that glucose from the blood and use it for

---

* In rats, it's called the diestrus phase.

energy or store it for future use. This process helps maintain stable blood-sugar levels, ensuring that cells get the energy they need while preventing excessive blood sugar, which can lead to health problems like diabetes and nuisance problems like food cravings. But during the luteal phase, insulin is less sensitive to glucose, leading to sharper increases and decreases in blood sugar that can make us hungry and cranky, and lead us to crave more food.

I have observed these differences in my own body when wearing a continuous blood glucose monitor,[*] which I do periodically to learn more about how my body responds to food. I saw very distinct differences in peaks and valleys in my blood-glucose levels, created from eating carbohydrate-rich foods, depending on my cycle phase. Eating a sweet potato in the follicular phase gave me a moderate increase in blood glucose levels (an increase of approximately 25 mg/dL), whereas eating the exact same thing in the luteal phase led to a blood glucose spike almost double that. And because what goes up must come down, the blood glucose crash I got from eating the sweet potato in the luteal phase was steeper than the one I'd experienced in the follicular phase. This is something that is known to prompt hunger and food cravings (and I can confirm that for me it does). This is nothing unique to sweet potatoes and nothing unique to me. Women experience higher highs and lower lows in the luteal phase than the follicular, contributing to the greater hunger that many women report in the luteal phase.

Although these changes can feel annoying, they are purposeful. These are just some of the switches that progesterone flips to ensure that our bodies are doing the things they need to do to support a pregnancy. But you can see how this is at odds with the one-size-fits-all nu-

---

[*] If you are interested in learning more about blood glucose fluctuations, what causes them, and their impact on health, I highly recommend you follow the Glucose Goddess on Instagram (or get one of her wonderful books). She has a ton of great resources (and fun graphics) to acquaint you with how to avoid what she calls "riding the glucose roller coaster," which is when your blood-glucose levels go sky high and then crash, making you hungrier and crankier.

tritional advice most of us get that tells us to eat a certain number of calories each day, regardless of our hormonal state. Most women are never taught that it is normal to feel hungrier and need more food in the last two weeks of the cycle than the first. This mismatch between what we are told by experts and what our bodies are trying to tell us conditions us to ignore our body's signals. It creates an environment in which women are all but guaranteed to develop an adversarial relationship with their bodies and hunger. *Especially* in the luteal phase.

It is absolutely no coincidence that research finds that food craving, binge eating, disordered eating, and emotional eating all reach their peak in the luteal phase. Because when we don't give our bodies the nourishment they need—especially when they are preparing for something as evolutionarily consequential as pregnancy—our bodies will push back. And often this pushback can lead us to eat far less nutritious food than what we would have eaten if we had just listened to our hunger in the first place. It creates preoccupation with food, frustration with ourselves for "overeating," and irritability from the stress of not having our biological needs met. And because the only set of nutrition guidelines we've ever been given is one that wasn't designed for female bodies, we think that *we're* the problem. We think *"If only I had better self-control"* or *"Why is my body betraying me?"* How many hours have each of us spent shaming ourselves for not being able to follow nutrition rules that weren't made for us?

Understanding our bodies' needs in the luteal phase—and honoring them—has the potential to dramatically improve our relationship with food and, ultimately, with ourselves. It can help us begin to dismantle the harmful self-narratives many of us have about being untrustworthy and lacking in self-control when it comes to food. And this is good for us in so many ways. It is good for our physical health. It is good for our emotional state. And it is good for helping to repair the damaged relationship so many of us have with our appetites and eating behavior.

Learning to listen to our bodies and trust our hunger is also good for fertility and our hormonal health. Because female mammals—including humans—will turn ovulation off like a light switch if the brain gets the sense that energy intake won't be plentiful enough to pull off a successful pregnancy. Food intake is the single most powerful factor affecting female fertility that has ever been identified (*ever identified!!*), because female bodies want nothing to do with initiating pregnancies that are unlikely to make it to the finish line. For women, eating is about far more than simply providing nourishment to the body. It also provides the brain with information about the availability of resources in the current environment.

A COOL THING ABOUT FEMALE BODY FAT

Although women sometimes lament the fact that their bodies love to create fat stores around their butt and thighs, our bodies like to store fat there for a reason. This fat—called gluteofemoral fat—is where our bodies stockpile long-chain polyunsaturated fatty acids like docosahexaenoic acid (DHA), which are critical for fueling neonatal brain development. Long-chain fatty acids make up about 20 percent of the dry weight of the human brain, making them something developing babies need a lot of. And because babies need more of these fats than we can take in from the food we eat (research using isotope-labeled fatty acids shows that 60–80 percent of the long-chain fatty acids in human breast milk come from maternal fat stores rather than a mother's current dietary intake), our bodies stockpile them on our butts and thighs throughout our reproductive years to ensure ready access when we need them.

Successful pregnancies require not just having enough calories; they also require that we have enough fat. This is yet another reason why the luteal phase ushers in a season of eating (and why ovulation tends to get disrupted when body fat is too low). Regularly experiencing a cycle phase characterized by increased rest and food intake has helped women put on and maintain the critical fat stores necessary for pregnancy and lactation even in the face of food shortfalls.

When we get enough food and eat regularly, it tells our brain that we have access to resources and that a pregnancy could likely be supported. And under these conditions, we ovulate and produce sex hormones. Conversely, when we don't get enough food or don't eat regularly, it tells our brain that resources are scarce and pregnancy might be a bad idea. Under these conditions, we are less likely to ovulate and produce sex hormones.* This is why there was a 66 percent decline in births during the Dutch famine in the Second World War. This is also why fasting, calorie restriction, and intense exercise† without increasing calorie intake—while fine for men—can wreak havoc on female fertility and sex hormone production. Pregnancy is so energy demanding and costly to women that our bodies won't roll the dice by allowing an egg to be released unless there is a good chance we'd be able to finish what we start if fertilization occurs.

I encourage you to unlearn the traditional rules of one-size-fits-all nutrition and learn to get in tune with your hunger. Our ancestors survived for millions of years without nutrition labels or government-mandated food pyramids, so our bodies are a lot smarter about food than many of us give them credit for. Learning to listen to your hunger and giving your body the food you need in the luteal phase can do a huge world of good when it comes to improving your relationship with food. While it's true that our hunger can lead us astray when we are eating processed foods (which are engineered to increase our

---

* Well, it's not that we don't produce *any* sex hormones. We just produce a lot less of them. Most of our estrogen and almost all our progesterone is produced in the ovaries from the process of ovulation.

† Although it used to be thought that female athletes would develop amenorrhea because they were simply exercising too hard, research by Dr. Jerilynn Prior and others have found that exercise isn't the issue at all. Instead, female athletes who develop amenorrhea do so because they are not taking in enough calories to offset their increased energy expenditure from heavy exercise. Female athletes who take in enough calories to offset what they're burning maintain healthy cycles. So don't be afraid to push yourself as an athlete because you're afraid of losing your cycle. Instead, double down on your efforts to make sure that you are providing your body with enough calories to outpace what is being burned when you train.

hunger as we eat them . . . the exact opposite of what real food does), when we eat whole, minimally processed foods, hunger is a guide that contains millions of years of inherited wisdom from our ancestors. Listening to our bodies and feeding them what they need in the luteal phase is a step in the right direction to feeling significantly better during this phase.

Fitness, Resistance Training, and How to Exercise Like a Girl

The big takeaway from this chapter is that one-size-fits-all health and wellness advice doesn't work for women. And nutrition is just part of the story. There are also cycle-based differences in how we respond to exercise that most of us haven't been told about. Which means that some of the time we spend sweating at the gym may not have the effect we want it to. When you have a body that is hard at work preparing for pregnancy, it's going to have fewer resources left over for doing things like building strength and fueling intense cardio sessions.

For example, in one study, researchers looked at whether women's ability to put on lean muscle mass and build strength from resistance training differed across the cycle. To test this, they had two groups of women cyclically alternate between high- and low-frequency strength-training sessions over the course of twelve weeks (which is the equivalent of three menstrual cycles). During the high-frequency weeks, women did leg-based strength training four times a week. During low-frequency weeks, women did this training two times a week. Half of the women did the high-frequency training during the follicular phase and the low-frequency training during the luteal phase. The other half did the opposite (high-frequency training during the luteal phase and low-frequency during the follicular). At the end of the study period, all the women had spent six weeks doing high-frequency strength training and six weeks doing low-frequency strength training.

CYCLE PHASE-BASED STRENGTH GAINS

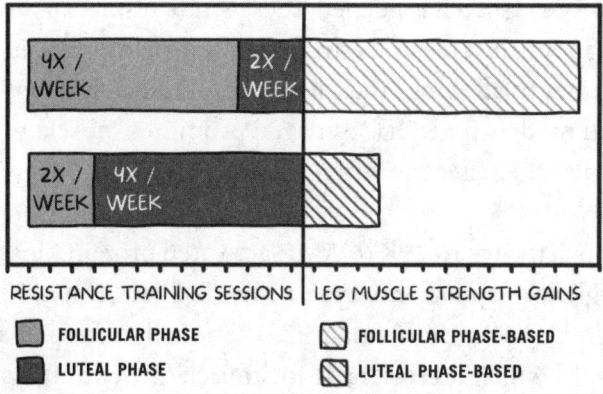

Now, if a day-is-a-day-is-a-day in the world of women's resistance training and weight lifting, the researchers should have found that the two groups of women each put on equal amounts of muscle mass from their leg-based strength training. But this isn't what the researchers found at all. The cycle phase mattered in women's strength gains. And it mattered quite a bit. You can see the results in the figure above. When the high-frequency training period was done during the estrogenic follicular phase, women's leg strength increased 40 percent compared to where it was prior to training. But when the high-frequency portion of their training took place in the progesterone-a-rific luteal phase, the exact same amount of exercise yielded only a 27 percent increase in muscle strength. These women got 13 percent lower gains in strength just because they did most of their training in the luteal phase.

This pattern isn't unique to one study. Other research using a similar design found that women doing high-frequency strength training in the follicular phase saw a 32 percent increase in muscle mass, while those training in the luteal phase only saw a 13 percent increase. Even more frustrating, some studies have found that women doing high-intensity training in the luteal phase actually experienced a *decrease* in strength, compared to gains seen during the follicular phase—which seems completely unfair.

While more research is needed, these study results align with what we know about the roles of estrogen and progesterone in the body when it comes to all things muscle growth. Research in both humans and animal models finds that estrogen promotes muscle growth and repair, while progesterone often does the opposite. Here's how it works.

Estrogen activates AMPK (5'AMP-activated protein kinase), which enhances glucose uptake into type 1 muscle fibers, improving muscle function and exercise performance. Additionally, estrogen stimulates satellite cells, which are essential for muscle growth. It also inhibits protein breakdown in existing muscle tissue and boosts growth hormone release in response to exercise, promoting new muscle formation. Essentially, estrogen prepares our bodies to gain strength from resistance training, making the follicular phase—especially near ovulation when estrogen levels peak—a prime time for building strength.

Progesterone, on the other hand, does none of these things. And some of the things that it does are downright antagonistic to strength building. For example, progesterone suppresses the release of growth hormone (bad for muscle growth), prevents glucose uptake into muscle fibers (bad for muscle performance), and is catabolic (meaning it breaks down tissues instead of building them up). And although these sorts of actions might be great in the context of preparing the body for pregnancy (and, as far as evolution is concerned, there is no higher calling than that), they're not terribly helpful when you're trying to build muscle. And when you couple these strength-antagonizing tendencies with the fact that strength-building testosterone takes a nose dive during the luteal phase, you can pretty much kiss the hopes of equal-returns-for-equal-workouts goodbye.

For all these reasons, your luteal and follicular phase are not equivalent when it comes to building strength. Your body is less able to go full tilt on strength building during the luteal phase, which means that any investment you make in strength training at this time is likely going to have less of a payoff than the same investment made just a few weeks later.

Progesterone can also affect our performance *during* workouts. Research suggests that progesterone may reduce strength and power during exercise and increase the level of strain we feel during activities like running or taking a spin class. This can have the effect of making exercise feel less fun for us in the luteal phase than the follicular and may impair our performance.

For example, research finds that progesterone can affect how energetic and powerful we feel during exercise. This is because progesterone levels increase fatigue and reduce muscle activation in ways that can make us feel weaker and impact performance. Additionally, progesterone can influence muscle recovery and repair processes that occur during exercise in ways that may impair overall performance. These changes—especially when coupled with luteal phase changes in temperature, metabolism, and respiratory drive—can make high-intensity workouts feel more strenuous in the luteal phase than in the follicular phase. We become more easily overheated and winded in the luteal phase* than the follicular.

The net effect of all this is that exercise can feel less fun and more depleting to us in the luteal phase than the follicular. And this is an idea that, while still new, has some research support. In one study, for example, researchers measured women's perceived strain from endurance training they completed in both the luteal and follicular phases of the cycle. What they found was that the same fifty minutes of

---

* When I learned this, a serious light bulb went off in my head. I have always had days at the gym when I feel like I am out of breath. The way I described it to my doctor was that it felt like I had a hole in my heart that was preventing my blood from getting oxygenated enough. We weren't able to figure out what was going on, so I set it aside until I came across a paper on respiratory drive across the cycle and everything clicked into place. Since that time, I have tracked these episodes and—sure enough—they map onto peak progesterone across my cycle. Sometimes, these effects are significant enough to make me get short of breath even when doing public speaking. We will return to this issue in the next chapter when we talk about premenstrual exacerbation (PME) of asthma.

endurance training felt significantly more difficult for them in the luteal phase than follicular. Other research finds that these cycle-phase-based patterns are particularly pronounced when women exercise in warm temperatures, since their already elevated body temperatures can make it harder to cool off.

Together, this research suggests that women may benefit from adjusting their workouts in ways that take their cyclically changing sex hormones into account. Although there is still a lot of research to be done in this area (and recent research reviews highlight the fact the things we know are far outnumbered by the things we don't), the available evidence suggests that there may be little to lose and a lot to gain from adjusting our workouts to (a) maximize strength building and intense cardiovascular work in the follicular phase, and (b) prioritize lower-impact, more restorative work in the luteal. While the research in this area isn't yet conclusive, I can point to two pieces of evidence that suggest it could be effective.

The first is from a research study I recently conducted with 28 Wellness looking at the effects of their cycle-based exercise program on women's fitness gains and body satisfaction. We made comparisons between naturally cycling women who exercise regularly in a way that is tailored to their cycle phase (doing high-intensity exercise and resistance training in the follicular phase and more restorative work in their luteal phase) and those who exercise regularly but do not change the type of exercise they do based on their cycle phase. We made comparisons between the two groups of women on things like energy levels, fitness, food craving, and satisfaction with the look and feel of their bodies.

There were clear differences in how the two groups felt when it came to all things health, wellness, and body satisfaction. The women who were exercising in tune with their cycles felt healthier, happier, more energetic, more satisfied with the look and feel of their bodies, sexier, and more physically fit than the women exercising the old-fashioned way. They also reported having fewer food cravings, more control over their eating, and better mental health than the other group. These changes (along with a whole host of other positive changes, including more menstrual cycle regularity and greater control over their period symptoms) suggest that honoring our body's distinct fitness needs in the luteal phase may pay dividends.

The second piece of evidence I offer you is my personal experience incorporating a cycle-based approach to my fitness practice. And while this is not a carefully controlled research study, it is still data. Adopting a cycle-based approach to my exercise has been a game changer for my relationship with exercise and my body.

Like most people I know, I used to do the same series of workouts every week regardless of my hormonal state. And although I felt reasonably satisfied with my level of fitness, there was a lot about the process of staying fit that felt miserable to me. *Especially* in the luteal phase. I'd tire more easily, I couldn't lift my maximum during resistance training, and often—once I was done at the gym and ready to start my day—rather than feeling energized, I'd feel completely depleted and like I needed to take a nap.

Although I knew what was going on hormonally thanks to my research, it took me years to abandon the practice of doing the same workout every week. I was afraid that I would get weaker or lose the muscle tone that I'd worked so hard to build over the years.

But one day, after a particularly unpleasant week at the gym, I decided that I was finally ready to put all the science I'd been reading to the test. And I would try doing a six-month quasi experiment on myself to see if changing my workouts to be more in tune with my cycles would allow me to maintain my current level of fitness. In particular, I changed things in a way that emphasized heavy resistance training and intense cardio in the follicular phase (when estrogen was flipping all the "grow muscle" and "be powerful" switches in my body) and then shifted to focus on lower-impact work in the luteal phase, when my body wasn't doing me any favors when it comes to building strength anyway.

During those six months—despite the fact that I did fewer lifting sessions than I had in the past—I got stronger. I began being able to lift heavier weights than I could prior to changing my workouts, and I could do it with less effort. This was a big breakthrough for me. And although I didn't get into a DEXA scanner to look at my body composition before and after making the switch (which would have been the more sciency way to do my self-experiment), it certainly didn't look like I'd lost any muscle mass and my clothes fit the same. Since these were the metrics that mattered to me (with strength being the big one), this was a huge victory and a turning point for me. And this is how I have been doing things ever since.

I feel healthier, and my luteal phase is less of a beatdown because I am respecting my body's differing needs at this time. This doesn't mean that I let my cycle totally run the show when it comes to physical activity. It just means that I use my effort wisely and take steps to avoid depleting myself unnecessarily in the luteal phase.

Exercising in a way that is mindful of my sex hormones has been hugely empowering for me. It may be for you too. This doesn't mean that you need to change anything about your gym routine if what you're doing works for you (as we say in Texas, if it ain't broke, don't fix it), but for those of you looking to change things up, consider emphasizing heavy resistance training (and high-intensity cardio) in the follicular and shifting to less strenuous forms of exercise in the luteal phase. If you're like me, you may get stronger and feel a whole lot better than you do now.

Things to Do Today to Harness Your Hormones for Optimal Fitness and Nutrition

Let me preface this section with the reminder that I am a researcher, not a medical doctor. If you think you might want to try any of the ideas below—especially if you have any preexisting medical conditions—have a chat with your health-care provider first. These are just ideas that you might want to consider incorporating into your nutrition and exercise practice based on the latest research.

- Start tracking the relationship between your cycle and all things fitness and nutrition. Tracking your hunger, food intake, energy levels, and exercise performance for a couple of months will give you important insight into how *your* body responds to hormonal changes (remember: each of us is a little different). You can use the tracking resources I have provided for you at the end of the book, a cycle-tracking app like 28, or a diary that you create on your own (the cycle-tracking resources at the end of the book can be used as a template for you to make a cycle-tracking map customized to you).

- Abandon the one-cycle-phase-fits-all nutritional guidelines we've all been force-fed* since childhood and repeat after me: *My body burns through energy faster in the luteal phase than the follicular, meaning I should listen to my body if it is telling me to eat more.* It's nonsensical for women with cycles to be told to maintain consistent calorie intake day in and day out. When we aim to eat the same number of calories each day regardless of what's going on with our hormones, it can make us tired, hungry, and cranky, and can trigger food cravings and binge-eating episodes when our body fights back and demands more. This doesn't mean you should grab a handful of Oreos after each meal to make sure you're getting enough calories in the luteal phase (processed foods will just make you hungrier). Instead, it means learning to trust your hunger and eat more when your body tells you what it needs. I'll give you some specific ideas about how to eat to support your cycle in chapter 11.
- Consider adding a little extra protein into your diet during the luteal phase to improve energy and minimize food cravings. The research behind this idea isn't rock solid just yet (very few people have asked the question), but the reasoning behind it is sound and it's a low-cost thing to try. The idea behind upping protein intake is that *maybe* we can curb hunger and diminish food cravings by helping replen-

---

* With me, the pun is always intended.

ish the amino acid stores that get depleted by progesterone as it fuels the pregnancy-preparation process.* And there is no better way to stock up on the amino acids your body needs for building projects than by eating high-quality protein. This can be animal protein (e.g., fish, eggs), plant protein (e.g., black beans, tempeh), or some combination of both. This is another practice that I have incorporated into my life. Although I have limited data to suggest that it is doing anything special in my body to help replenish amino acids, it definitely helps me feel fuller longer. You may want to consider adding a little extra protein into your diet during the luteal phase and see if it has the same effect for you.

Eating a higher protein diet in the luteal phase will also help you keep your blood-glucose levels more stable in ways that will help you feel less hungry all the time. This is especially true if you eat the protein (and vegetables!) at the beginning of a meal and the carbohydrate-dense foods last. Eating low-carbohydrate foods first helps minimize the impact of the carbohydrates that you do eat on blood-glucose levels, making you stay fuller longer. You can also check out the Glucose Goddess (www.glucosegoddess.com) for more easy-to-implement ideas on how to keep you blood-glucose levels more stable in the luteal phase.

- If you are not happy with your existing workout routine (or are looking to try something new), shake things up by adopting a hormonally aligned workout schedule. This can take whatever form you want it to, but research suggests that we can get the most bang for our buck if we emphasize resistance training and intense cardio sessions in the follicular phase and lower-impact, restorative work in the luteal phase. Before you get started, make note of your energy levels, mood, strength, and whatever other fit-

---

* This is just a hypothesis at this point, so take with the appropriate grain of salt.

ness metrics you're interested in beforehand. Then, make the switch. I would recommend sticking with it for a minimum of three months before drawing conclusions about whether it is working for you or not. Lasting change in the body takes time, so be patient. Make notes about what's getting better, what's getting worse, and make adjustments as you go.

- Be gentle with yourself in the luteal phase. This is a time when it's easier for us to overheat (because of our higher body temperature), it's harder for our bodies to recover (our heart rate is higher and our heart-rate variability is lower, making it more difficult for our body to fully unwind and recover at night when we sleep), and our energy needs are higher. Because of this, our bodies need more thoughtful, intentional care than they do in the follicular phase. This means that we need to be gentle with ourselves if we want to feel our best. During the luteal phase, make a special effort to prioritize going to bed early, drinking enough water, getting (low-impact or restorative) physical activity, limiting or abstaining from alcohol, eating healthy foods, and minimizing stress. Although doing these sorts of things is always good for us, we're less able to recover from momentary lapses in self-care in the luteal phase than we are in the follicular. For me, taking extra care in the luteal phase means going to bed earlier, doing things that feed my soul (long walks outside, journaling, reading for pleasure), being more inclined to pass on a glass of wine with dinner, and taking short (ten-to-twenty-minute) naps when my body tells me it needs one. Think about what this would look like for you and start putting these things into practice.

CHAPTER 9

FROM PMS TO PRIMARY CARE

*Mystery symptoms, mental health,
and premenstrual exacerbation of . . . everything*

Being a woman can sometimes feel like being a living, breathing medical mystery. A lot of times when our bodies do things that worry us, no one can give us a straight answer about why we feel that way. Whether it's suddenly feeling exhausted all the time, having pain that comes out of nowhere, or finding ourselves in the midst of an unexpected flare-up of a condition we thought we'd outgrown in childhood, we all know what it's like to be on the business end of a shoulder-shrug diagnosis (when you go to the doctor with a health-care concern and are given a shrug, some vague reassurances, and a suggestion that your symptoms are . . . drum roll, please . . . all in your head).

The truth is medicine just doesn't understand our bodies all that well. And the reason for this is largely because of the research bias we talked about in chapter 4. Doctors don't know everything there is to know about female bodies because research conducted on female bodies is the exception rather than the rule in most areas of medicine. And research is particularly lacking for the luteal phase. There isn't a whole lot of information out there about what our bodies are supposed to feel like or how they're likely to respond to treatments or medical interventions at this time because very few people are doing the research. This can make the luteal phase of the cycle a particularly vulnerable time for women, because it's a time in which our bodies are most likely to experience symptoms or side effects that no one has ever heard of before.

This is problematic because there is little reason to assume that the way our bodies respond to something in the follicular phase will be the same as the way it responds in the luteal. Progesterone affects our immune system, our metabolism, our circulatory system, our respiratory system, all our other hormones, and pretty much everything else that goes on with our bodies, inside and out. Everything changes in response to progesterone release. When everything we know about women's health is derived from research conducted on men or on women in the early follicular phase, it means that we're going to spend roughly half of our adult lives experiencing things that nobody has a good explanation for.

Fixing this problem is going to require that we completely overhaul the way women are handled as subjects in research science. And this is something I think is absolutely necessary if we are to have any hope of providing women with the same level of health care that we are able to offer men. In the meantime, though, there are things about yourself that you can learn in order to help better navigate the way you experience your body, your symptoms of illness, and your experiences with psychological or medical interventions in the luteal phase.

We're going to start this chapter talking about everything your doctor probably hasn't told you about your cycle and physical health. Because there is a lot about our health and our bodies that changes across the cycle. We will then talk about the way these changes across the cycle impact women's experiences of health and disorder in the luteal phase, including the very real possibility that our cycles might impact the way our bodies respond to medical interventions ranging from prescription drugs to psychotherapy. Lastly, we will talk about the health benefits of progesterone and its understudied therapeutic benefits . . . and why the future of medical research needs more hormonal balance.

From Bad to Worse: Chronic Conditions, Pain, and Luteal-Phase Worsening of Symptoms

The first thing we need to do is go over some of the physical changes that go on in our bodies in the luteal phase. And there are a lot of them because, as noted, pregnancy is a whole-body job. It requires the cooperation of every system our bodies have, making the effects of progesterone pervasive. But rather than spending paragraph after paragraph waxing scientific about all the bits, pieces, and nanoparticles that rise and fall in the luteal phase, I am going to give you a nice, succinct bullet-point list of those that are most relevant to our discussion here. So here they are, in no particular order:

- **Changes in pain perception.** Progesterone affects pain perception in ways that can make pain more noticeable and less tolerable in the luteal phase than the follicular.* Progesterone does this by changing the activities of neuropeptides like substance P (a neuropeptide involved in pain transmission . . . P for pain) and neurotransmitters like GABA, glutamate, dopamine, serotonin, and norepinephrine. Although this is something that makes a whole lot of sense when we consider that pain is something we experience to keep our body safe from harm (and as far as evolution is concerned, there's no better time to make sure

---

* Interestingly, the results of research on cycle-based effects of pain perception is somewhat mixed, suggesting that the impact of our hormones on how we feel is likely to be nuanced and condition-specific. For example, although many conditions feel worse in the luteal phase than the follicular, research finds that pain from temporomandibular joint (TMJ) dysfunction and migraine seem to be lower in the luteal phase than the follicular.

that your body is safe from harm than when pregnant or preparing to be), it can lead to reduced pain tolerance and a greater reliance on nonprescription pain relievers in the luteal phase compared to the follicular.*

- **Changes in the immune system.** We've talked about this one already, but here is a quick review. Because progesterone is charged with making the body a safe place for pregnancy, it causes changes in the immune system that make it tolerant to embryos. It does this by downregulating facets of the immune system that promote inflammation and upregulating aspects of the immune system that promote immunological tolerance. Although this progesterone-fueled immunological tinkering isn't something that most of us notice, it can have a big impact on how you feel if you suffer from an autoimmune disease. For example, for diseases like lupus and multiple sclerosis (MS)†—which are caused by cells involved in the immune response that gets heightened in response to progesterone—the luteal phase makes symptoms worse (about 80 percent of lupus flare-ups occur in the luteal phase). Conversely, autoimmune diseases fueled by the arm of the immune system that gets quieted in response to progesterone tend to get better. For example, women with rheumatoid arthritis (RA) experience fewer symptoms in the luteal phase than the follicular, and about 75 percent of sufferers experience complete remission during pregnancy because it is a high-progesterone state.
- **Relaxation of our smooth muscles.** Progesterone has been shown to have a relaxing effect on smooth muscles

---

* Because pain tolerance varies across the cycle, the exact same symptoms may be experienced at different levels of intensity depending on what women's hormones are doing at the time. This is yet another reason that women should be tested as research subjects in both the follicular and luteal phases of the cycle.

† Although MS is also impacted by misbehavior from cells involved in our cell-mediated immune response.

in the digestive system, slowing gut motility. This has the effect of increasing nutrient absorption, which is great for pregnancy, but can make irritable bowel syndrome (IBS) worse by creating more uncomfortable backups than usual.

- **Changes in neurotransmission that (a) increase threat perception and (b) dampen pleasure.** As we discussed in chapter 6, because progesterone is getting our bodies ready for pregnancy, it shifts our perception in ways that make the world seem simultaneously more dangerous and less promising of pleasure than it does in the follicular phase. And while this serves an important function (keeping us safe and preventing us from wasting our limited energy on unnecessary pursuits when we're preparing to have a baby on board), it can pour gasoline on the fire of mental health struggles.
- **Metabolic changes.** Our metabolism revs up in the luteal phase, which can make us hungrier. And when this hunger isn't honored because we've been taught a one-size-fits-all version of what energy needs are supposed to look like, it can trigger binge-eating episodes as well as bulimia. It may also change the rate at which our bodies metabolize medications, potentially changing their latency of action and efficacy.
- **Changes in respiratory drive.** Progesterone increases respiratory drive, which is our urge to breathe. Progesterone acts on the respiratory centers in the brain (particularly in the medulla), enhancing their sensitivity to carbon dioxide (CO_2). This makes the body more responsive to higher CO_2 levels, causing it to work harder to expel it more efficiently. As a result, women tend to breathe more frequently and deeply during the luteal phase, which can cause feelings of breathlessness. Progesterone does this to maintain proper acid-base balance in the body and ensure that enough oxygen is delivered to tissues in the face of our heightened metabolic demands.

As you can see, progesterone initiates a huge range of changes in the body that can have a very powerful effect on how we feel. This means that the symptoms of chronic conditions we have and even the ways we respond to the treatments we've been given can change across the cycle too. And there is a growing body of research suggesting that this very much might be the case. Many of women's health problems—both physical and mental—can become worse in the luteal phase than the follicular, an effect that's known as premenstrual* exacerbation (PME). When women aren't told about these effects, they can create unnecessary anxiety and the need for doctors' appointments that could potentially be avoided if we understood our cycle better.

Consider Ava's story. Ava is a twenty-nine-year-old school guidance counselor who developed asthma in her late teenage years. Her symptoms were relatively mild until she moved to the city in her mid-twenties to start graduate school, when her symptoms started worsening on and off in ways that set off her internal alarm bells:

> I felt like my breathing had gotten worse, so I scheduled a doctor's appointment for late the following week to have it looked at. When I got there, my breathing test came back normal (for me), and I was feeling a little better, so I left and thought things must be getting better. Flash-forward another couple of weeks, and it happened again. So I scheduled another doctor appointment for the following week and the same thing happened. This same thing happened two more times over the next three years before I saw something on my social media feed from IAPMD† about how asthma can get worse in the luteal phase. After that,

---

* Note that "premenstrual" is being broadly construed here. Researchers use this term to describe anything ranging from a couple of days before our periods start to the entirety of the luteal phase (and everything in between). This lack of precision makes the literature on PME pretty messy since some people are studying the entire length of the luteal phase, whereas others are only studying the late luteal phase. Importantly, both can be related to worsening of symptoms.
† International Association for Premenstrual Disorders.

I was able to connect the dots. I started tracking my cycle and saw that, lo and behold, my asthma was getting worse after I ovulated. I went back to my doctor with information about premenstrual worsening of asthma and we were able to get me additional treatments to take after ovulation. It's been so helpful and a huge relief to know that this is really common and nothing serious. It's also been hugely helpful to have additional treatment support during times when my breathing feels so labored. I was afraid that my asthma was getting worse. Or that it had transformed into something much, much worse.

Ava is far from alone in experiencing physical symptoms that change across the cycle. Almost half of asthmatic women report that their symptoms get worse in the luteal phase compared to the follicular. And asthma is far from being unusual in this way. Research finds that health conditions including asthma, migraine, eczema, chronic fatigue syndrome, fibromyalgia, bladder pain, epilepsy, IBS, lupus, MS, and diabetes can all have symptoms that get worse in the luteal phase compared to the follicular. Although the specific mechanisms responsible for this differ, the effect is the same: luteal-phase worsening of symptoms due to predictably occurring biological changes that women are never told about.

WHY AM I SO BLOATED IN THE LUTEAL PHASE?

In my conversations with women about things that make them crazy during the luteal phase, water retention and bloating are two that I frequently hear about. And the reason these are such common "hormonal" experiences for us is because estrogen and progesterone both play important roles in our body's electrolyte balance (particularly the balance of sodium and potassium) and gut motility. When our hormones go through big changes like they do in the luteal phase, our electrolyte balance can get out of sync and our gut can slow down in ways that make us feel . . . *ugggghhhh.*

> If you feel bloated in the luteal phase, here are a few things that research suggests can help. **If your problem is water retention**, consider reducing sodium intake, staying hydrated (your body holds on to water when it's dehydrated), exercising regularly (your body gets better at maintaining electrolyte balance when fit), or taking vitamin B_6 (it enhances kidney function and has mild diuretic properties). **If your problem is a slow-moving gut**, the answer is increasing your fiber intake (by eating a diet rich in fruits, veggies, and whole grains), exercising (moving your muscles helps move things along, so to speak), and drinking plenty of water.

Research finds that certain mental health symptoms can also worsen considerably in the luteal phase. Symptoms of depression, obsessive-compulsive disorder (OCD), bipolar disorder, posttraumatic stress disorder (PTSD), eating disorders, panic disorder, and schizophrenia* often worsen in the last two weeks of the cycle compared to the first. Studies show that almost 70 percent (!) of women with major depressive disorder and bipolar disorder experience PME of psychological symptoms. And among those with bulimia, the frequency of binge-eating episodes increases an average of 60 percent in the luteal phase.

Unfortunately, we're never told about this worsening of various symptoms or conditions in the luteal phase, or the idea that it can be normal for women. Because of this, many women who suffer from PME, like Ava, assume that their condition must be getting worse. Or that there must be something far more serious and troubling going on. This can prompt a lot of unnecessary doctor visits and symptom-googling.

---

* It's important to note that these changes in mental health are distinct from severe PMS or PMDD. PME of mental health disorders is when you have issues that manifest during the follicular phase and worsen in the luteal, whereas women with severe PMS or PMDD are asymptomatic during the first half of the cycle.

COMMON MEDICAL AND PSYCHOLOGICAL CONDITIONS
EXACERBATED BY PROGESTERONE

MEDICAL CONDITIONS
Acne
Acute appendicitis
Acute intermittent porphyria
Aphthous ulcers
Asthma
Diabetes
Endocrine allergy and anaphylaxis
Epilepsy
Erythema multiforme
Glaucoma
Hereditary angioedema
Irritable bowel syndrome
Migraine
Multiple sclerosis
Paroxysmal supraventricular tachycardia
Rheumatoid arthritis
Urticaria

PSYCHOLOGICAL CONDITIONS
Anxiety
Bipolar disorder
Eating disorders
Menopausal transition-related depression
Premenstrual dysphoric disorder

Thankfully, this can be a thing of the past for you now. Above is a list of chronic health conditions for which PME is frequently documented. Note that this isn't an exhaustive list. PME is still a relatively new "diagnosis," and researchers are learning more about it every day. If you have a chronic health condition, tracking your symptoms across the cycle will help you learn whether your condition is affected by your changing sex hormones.

Learning whether your symptoms vary across the cycle can be an important first step toward feeling how you want to more of the time, empowering you to take the necessary steps to call in additional reinforcements during times when you're most vulnerable to flare-ups. It can also create lasting peace of mind about the state of your health.

Beyond PME: Your Cycle and Clinical Outcomes

Given the existence of things like PME, PMS, and all of the other P words that regularly make women miserable in the luteal phase, it's pretty clear that progesterone's effects on the body are powerful and widespread. The implications of this truth are profound. Because if we recognize progesterone's cascading effects on systems in the body from head to toe, it means recognizing that it's possible that the way female bodies respond to medical interventions ranging from prescription drugs to surgery could differ depending on cycle phase.

And they very well may.

Although this is an idea that's woefully underresearched (a constant refrain in women's health), there is some evidence that women's clinical responses to medical interventions of all sorts may vary across the cycle. When it comes to prescription drugs, for example, the hormonal changes we experience across the cycle affect many of the mechanisms that impact how drugs are distributed, metabolized, absorbed, and excreted from the body. This means that a prescription drug that we take in the follicular phase may affect our body differently in the luteal phase.

For instance, studies show that progesterone affects both phase I (oxidation, reduction, hydrolysis) and phase II (conjugation) of drug metabolism processes in the body. These changes can affect a drug's efficacy, how it is broken down and excreted, and how long its effects last. Further, progesterone's slowdown effects on smooth muscle tissue and gastrointestinal (GI) motility could potentially exacerbate these differences by causing delayed or inconsistent uptake in the luteal phase compared to the follicular.

There are also cycle-based differences in blood pressure and plasma protein levels that may have important implications for the way women's bodies respond to drugs. For example, progesterone increases blood pressure, which can affect the rate at which drugs get diffused throughout the body. This can change how long it takes a drug to start working, how long it stays in circulation, and how effective it is. Progesterone is also known to impact levels of some of the plasma proteins that drugs bind to for transport in the bloodstream. These changes can affect the active concentration of drugs in the body, further affecting their effectiveness, toxicity, and side-effect profile.

Although there is almost no research dedicated to examining hormonally mediated differences in how women's bodies respond to drugs, there is some evidence that suggests that such effects may occur for at least some medications. For example, research finds that women's responses to both caffeine and theophylline (a medication used to manage asthma and COPD) seem to differ across the cycle. Both are metabolized more slowly in the luteal phase than the follicular, which means that the exact same cup of coffee and dose of medication will produce longer-lasting effects during the last two weeks of your cycle than the first. Researchers have also noted that women's responses to psychiatric medications like antipsychotics and antidepressants also vary over the cycle, but in opposite ways. They seem to be metabolized more quickly. For example, one recent research review found that women's blood levels of lithium (the drug commonly used to treat mania and bipolar disorder) were significantly lower in the luteal phase compared to the follicular phase, corresponding to premenstrual worsening of their symptoms. Other research found that increasing lithium doses during the luteal phase can help compensate for these declines, decreasing women's symptoms to pre-luteal-phase levels.

Although studies such as these suggest that taking a cycle-based approach to medication may be a promising pathway for improving women's ability to manage symptoms across the cycle (particularly in the face of premenstrual worsening of symptoms, at least some of which are likely to be caused by changes in how medications are metabolized), there is very little research on this topic. Almost no one is bothering to ask the question of whether women's hormones matter when it comes to how they respond to drugs because it is so much easier to assume that they don't.*

This should be unacceptable. The untested assumption that our bodies will respond to medication the same way in the luteal phase as they do in the follicular is hard to defend when you consider that progesterone has important effects on many of the processes our bodies use to metabolize and circulate drugs. Although it is likely that these responses will be similar enough across the cycle that we won't notice them some of the time, it is unlikely that this will be true *all* the time. Until we invest in understanding these cycle-based differences, women will be left navigating their health care on their own with incomplete information about what to expect from their medication, potentially compromising their treatment outcomes and leaving them vulnerable to unnecessary side effects.

The fact is, as our hormones change, our bodies change. This means that any response that our body gives us from any intervention or therapy we might introduce will differ depending on what's going on with our primary sex hormones. And this is true whether the intervention is a medication, psychotherapy, or even surgery or vaccinations.

Research finds that women's sex hormones impact a variety of systems in the body that can have an impact on our ability to be sedated for, and recover from, surgery. Because progesterone and its metabolites have sedative effects, researchers have suggested that women's anesthesia needs may be lower in the luteal phase compared to the follicular. And because progesterone dampens the acute inflammatory response needed for effective wound healing and tissue repair, it

---

* To add my own anecdote here, I learned the hard way that I cannot take antihistamines like Benadryl in the luteal phase. Although they always make me tired, taking them in the luteal phase knocks me on my a** completely. The first time this happened, I fell asleep at the dinner table and stayed there for several hours before my boyfriend at the time was able to get me into my bed. The second time I did this (because I wanted to test whether it was a fluke), I fell asleep on the couch and was completely unrousable for ten hours.

may impact the ability of the body to recover from surgical interventions. Progesterone's effects on the immune system could also potentially impact our body's ability to create antibodies to vaccinations. And although the goodness or badness of this effect is hard to know, it is likely to be *different*.

In addition to influencing physical responses to medical treatments, such as medication, surgery, and vaccinations, sex hormones may also play a notable role in shaping how women respond to psychological interventions. Memory consolidation across the cycle is at its best when estrogen is high and at its worst when progesterone is high. Because of this, forms of psychotherapy that require memory consolidation to be effective may be less successful in the luteal phase than the follicular. And there is new research that suggests this just might be the case. It finds that exposure therapy for women with PTSD—a form of therapy that requires the brain to remember new, nonfearful associations with things that people are afraid of—is less effective at times in the cycle when progesterone is high than it is when progesterone is low. This suggests that women may get more bang for their buck out of exposure therapy sessions scheduled during the first two weeks of their cycle than they would for those scheduled during the last two weeks. It also suggests that women needing intensive treatment throughout the cycle may even benefit from the short-term use of progesterone-blocking drugs like mifepristone to improve their therapeutic outcomes.

There are so, *so* many potentially important research questions that haven't been addressed when it comes to cycle phase, progesterone, and health. Unfortunately, there are very few biomedical researchers who are doing the research required to know the extent to which cycle phase matters for clinical outcomes. It is my hope that this book (and the work being done by my amazing peers, who are pushing for cycle-informed research and clinical practice) begins the conversations necessary for this to change, and that we alter research practice to require that researchers design studies that start with the assumption that (a) there may be meaningful differences in how men and women respond to treatments, and (b) there may be meaningful differences in how women respond to treatments depending on cycle phase. Until we get to this point, what we know about women's health will remain woefully incomplete.

Progesterone for Health and a Plea for Hormonal Equity

Since we're here talking about how progesterone can affect how our bodies feel, I would be chagrined not to take a few minutes to talk about the health benefits of progesterone. I'm going to talk to you about these things not as a medical doctor (because I'm not one), but as a researcher. As someone who's spent a lot of time doing research on hormones, I'm shocked by the fact that progesterone hasn't gotten more attention from those in science and medicine because of all the amazing things it does for our bodies. Here is a quick laundry list of some of the ways that progesterone helps to support our health:

1. **Bone health:** Progesterone helps to maintain bone density and strength by stimulating the activity of osteoblasts, which are the cells responsible for building new bone tissue.
2. **Brain health:** Progesterone has calming, neuroprotective effects on the brain. It acts as a natural sedative, prevents brain damage from traumatic brain injuries, and may help protect against neurodegenerative diseases like Alzheimer's disease.
3. **Cardiovascular health:** Progesterone has cardiovascular benefits, including vasodilation (widening of the blood vessels), and may reduce the risk of cardiovascular disease and atherosclerosis (the formation of plaques on the walls of our arteries).
4. **Skin health:** Progesterone helps maintain skin elasticity and moisture, reducing the appearance of wrinkles. It may also help protect against the effects of UV radiation and oxidative stress on the skin.

5. **Anti-inflammatory properties:** Progesterone shifts the body into an anti-inflammatory state. This can help minimize the risk of developing certain autoimmune diseases as well as heart disease and other diseases of aging.*
6. **Relief during perimenopause:** Many of the terrible experiences women have during the early stages of perimenopause are the result of progesterone decreasing. When this happens, estrogen runs unopposed the full length of the cycle,† which can contribute to irritability, insomnia, hot flashes, loss of skin elasticity, and hair loss. Research finds that progesterone therapy in menopause is just as effective as estrogen in combating many of these symptoms *and*, unlike estrogen, it doesn't have any cardiovascular risks.
7. **Balancing the effects of estrogen:** Progesterone plays a crucial role in balancing the effects of estrogen within the body, a relationship that is essential for health, mood regulation, and cell growth. Estrogen and progesterone work together to regulate the menstrual cycle. Estrogen primarily promotes the growth and thickening of the endometrial lining of the uterus during the first half of the cycle. Progesterone then counters this effect by signaling the endometrial lining to stop growing and start differentiating or maturing, reducing the risk of endometriosis and cancer. A similar partnership between these two hormones is seen

---

* In fact, one of the things I've never been able to figure out is why there isn't more research into the possibility of using micronized progesterone for women on hormonal birth control who are at risk of developing the types of autoimmune disease known to be controlled by progesterone. I specify hormonal birth control users because (a) hormonal birth control does not contain progesterone, and (b) taking micronized progesterone across the cycle can suppress ovulation in natural cyclers.

† One of my favorite descriptions of what it is like when this happens comes from Lara Briden in her wonderful book *Hormone Repair Manual*. She describes estrogen as being like an eccentric friend you love spending time with for short intervals, but who can quickly become too much when you spend extended periods of time with her.

when we look at the growth and maintenance of breast tissue. Estrogen stimulates the growth of breast cells (which is why it can be linked with an increased breast cancer risk), whereas progesterone plays a role in the differentiation of these cells, which may reduce this risk. The two hormones work together as a yin and yang of cellular growth and excitability.

As you can see, there are a ton of health benefits to be had from progesterone, but most of us only hear about estrogen. Maybe it's because estrogen was discovered first, maybe it's because estrogen is just so sexy, maybe it's because the fake progesterone in birth control (progestins) makes us feel terrible and everyone assumes that progesterone does the same thing. Whatever the reason, this is a bias that has undoubtedly slowed the progress of women's health research. Because as of now, most researchers who study the effects of women's sex hormones on health outcomes usually only look at estrogen.

PROGESTERONE IS A SECRET WEAPON AGAINST ADDICTIVE BEHAVIORS

Progesterone is a potent ally in helping us quit behaviors that don't serve us, like drugs, alcohol, nicotine, and other addictive substances. Research conducted on animals and humans finds that progesterone decreases drug, alcohol, and nicotine cravings among those with addictions. It also decreases how rewarding and pleasurable addictive substances make our brains feel, making us less likely to become addicted to them in the first place. These changes are brought to you by progesterone-fueled increases in ALLO (which calms the brain by stimulating GABA receptors), and those changes in dopamine and serotonin signaling we talked about in chapter 6 that keep us safe at home instead of chasing costly rewards.

Interestingly, estrogen does the opposite. It fuels addiction

> by turning up the volume on our brain's responsiveness to rewards. This makes addictive substances more pleasurable and reinforcing in the follicular phase than the luteal phase. Although this isn't true for all rewards (food rewards are an exception), it is true for most.
>
> If you have a bad habit you want to quit, take advantage of this monthly superpower by scheduling your quit date in the luteal phase. Progesterone can help you solidify good habits for a couple of weeks before your next estrogen surge. And if you're on hormonal birth control and have a bad habit you want to quit, talk to your doctor about supplementing with micronized progesterone while in your quitting period. The progestins in hormonal birth control do not get converted into ALLO, so micronized progesterone may provide the same benefits of a natural cycle while also protecting yourself from pregnancy. Although this is not something that has yet been clinically tested (we are currently in the process of putting together a project to look at this), progesterone is low cost, safe, and has few side effects, so your care provider may be willing to let you try this off-label use in the name of better habits.

Despite all the beautifully neuroprotective benefits that progesterone provides the brain, almost *all* research on the neuroprotective effects of sex hormones on the development and progression of Alzheimer's disease looks exclusively at estrogen.[*] The same is true when

---

[*] Instead of including progesterone, much of the work on hormone therapy for menopause looks at the effects of estrogen plus a progestin, which isn't the same as progesterone. Progestins are mostly synthesized from testosterone and do not offer all the amazing health benefits of real-deal progesterone because they do not release ALLO when they are metabolized in the body. Most of the neuroprotective benefits of progesterone come from ALLO, and progesterone's anti-inflammatory effects are also not something you can get from progestins. So, even though there are some studies that give lip service to the fact that women have more than one

you look at the state of research on menopausal hormone therapy. The focus is usually on estrogen therapy or hormonal birth control. Progesterone almost never comes up.

My hope is that science and medicine will begin to invest as much time and energy into understanding the potential therapeutic benefits of progesterone as they have into understanding estrogen. I have little doubt that great inroads could be made into the prevention of diseases like Alzheimer's disease and conditions like chronic inflammation if researchers shifted their focus from estrogen only to a more balanced focus on estrogen and progesterone. Estrogen matters for women's mental and physical health, but progesterone matters too. Spread the word. The future of women's health care will be better for it.

Things You Can Do Today to Take Charge of Your Cyclically Changing Health

Although you have a somewhat shorter to-do list in this chapter compared to others, there are a few things that you can do today to help understand how the experiences of your body and your health change across the cycle:

- If you have a chronic illness (or unexplained pain that comes and goes), track your symptoms across the cycle. I'm sure you're getting tired of hearing me say "track your cycle, track your cycle . . ." over and over again, but I'm serious. Track your cycle! Tracking how you feel over the course of your cycle will help you better understand how your body responds to hormonal changes. This can be particularly helpful if you have a chronic condition or unexplained pain because it can help you learn what's worth

---

sex hormone, they are assuming that progestins are going to behave the same way as progesterone in the body, which simply isn't true.

getting alarmed about and what's not. It can also help you be more prepared so that you're never caught off guard by your health problems. I have learned a ton about the hormonal rhythm of my migraines (postovulation) and pain in my jaw from TMJ (late luteal). I have also learned that anything that might feel bad in my body (for example, if my ligaments feel sore from yoga) will invariably happen in the luteal phase. Knowing these things about myself tells me when I need to make sure I have my migraine medication handy and when I should and shouldn't get alarmed about new or worsening pain.

I think you'll find that learning your own biological rhythms can be incredibly comforting, and tracking our own rhythms can help us understand what matters for our body even though the research isn't there (yet).

- If you start a new daily medication, track your side effects for a full cycle. There is a chance that you could have new side effects pop up in one cycle phase but not the other because no one is required to test whether drugs interact with our sex hormones.* Tracking side effects will help you better understand reactions to any medications you take and whether there are any cycle-specific side effects that your doctor should be aware of. This is particularly important in the luteal phase, since whatever medication you're taking has probably never been tested on someone in the season of progesterone. Even though chances are everything will be fine (so no need to panic), note if there are unpleasant side effects that are specific to a given cycle phase. Talk to your doctor if you need to take additional steps to manage symptoms at times when side effects are worse.
- If you have a bad habit that you would like to quit (except for anything having to do with food intake), start in the luteal phase. Cutting out smoking, alcohol, caffeine, or other

---

* And because this isn't required, this isn't something most researchers do. ☹

drugs of abuse is going to be far easier in the luteal phase than the follicular. Take advantage of your progesterone-a-rific superpowers by using them to help make a positive change in your life. And if you are on birth control, you could even consider talking to your doctor about whether taking micronized progesterone might be a helpful tool in your recovery.*
- Support ovulation to support your health. Women are most likely to ovulate when they are healthy, nourished, safe, loved, and managing their stress effectively. We will talk in a more detailed way about how to support ovulation a little later in the book (see chapter 11).

Although health and health care are often assumed to be hormonally neutral, women's bodies don't work that way. The way we feel, the way we respond to illnesses, the way we respond to medications, the way we experience chronic conditions . . . *everything* is affected by our sex hormones. Unfortunately, medical research hasn't yet caught on to this fact. Until it does, it is up to each of us to understand how our bodies feel, how they respond to medication, and so on in the season of progesterone. It is my sincere hope that this book and the conversations it starts will act as catalysts changing the way medicine is done to better serve women. In the meantime, become an expert in your own body and an advocate for ensuring that your needs are met on all twenty-eight-ish days of your cycle.

---

* You probably do not want to use micronized progesterone if you are not on the pill or are postmenopausal because it will shut down your hypothalamic-pituitary-gonadal (HPG) axis and prevent your body from ovulating (unless you only take it after ovulation). Doing this for one or so cycles might not be all that bad for you, but I certainly wouldn't do this long term.

CHAPTER 10

WHEN A GOOD HORMONE GOES BAD

Answers and support for those with PMDD

So far we've been talking about all the wonderful, functional things that progesterone does to prepare our brains and bodies for pregnancy. Although some of these changes can create states of being that aren't necessarily our favorite things to experience, they usually serve a purpose. They keep us safe, sound, and prepared to manage the biological realities and demands of pregnancy.

PMDD, or premenstrual dysphoric disorder, isn't like that at all though. Rather than ushering in a time when women feel like a somewhat less exciting, less energetic, more sensitive version of themselves, for women with PMDD, the luteal phase ushers in what can feel like hell. They feel so anxious, depressed, angry, irritable, overwhelmed, and not like themselves that many consider ending their lives. They're less able to function at work, less able to function at home, and their relationships with themselves and others suffer. The worst part is that they feel this way every time they have a luteal phase, making PMDD a devastating diagnosis to get. None of us want to feel like we're living in hell roughly 50 percent of the time . . . particularly when the path to feeling better isn't always terribly clear.

Consider Grace's story. Grace is a twenty-two-year-old student who has been suffering from PMDD since the time she started her period at fourteen. Like a lot of women, Grace had a hard time getting a diagnosis because no one took her symptoms seriously. Despite feeling so depressed that she could barely get out of bed during the luteal phase, the first two doctors she consulted told her that her feelings were normal. She was told she just needed to get more sunlight or fresh air or decrease her stress. After several years of struggling to feel better on her own, she finally found a doctor who has taken her symptoms seriously and given her an accurate diagnosis. Nonetheless, finding a treatment she feels good about remains a struggle:

> I feel like PMDD has stolen my life from me. To me, progesterone is the devil. It's like, as soon as I ovulate, I know what's coming next, and it crushes me. It usually begins with me feeling overwhelmed by sadness and anger. This can make me lash out at people I care about. This hurts them and makes me feel like a monster. I know that I am driving people away, but it's like I can't help myself. Then it feels like everyone hates me and wishes I would go away.
>
> I have a hard time getting my schoolwork done at this time too. I just don't have motivation to do anything. So my performance at school suffers and I feel worthless and guilty about not being able to keep up. It makes me want to disappear or go away forever. And I know that the problem is my hormones. I feel better almost instantly when I get my period. It's then that I get a glimpse of what my life would be like if I was normal, which makes me happy and sad at the same time. I mean, it's great to feel good, but it's hard to feel happy when I know what's around the corner. It haunts me. My guess is that my body can't handle progesterone. So, I've been begging my doctor to give me a hysterectomy to make all of this end. He won't do it, so I have been looking for someone else who might. I don't want to be on the birth control pill again and antidepressants made me feel worse. It feels hopeless and there aren't a lot of solutions for women like me.

Grace is far from alone in feeling this way. Roughly 5 percent of women experience PMDD, a mood disorder that is specific to the luteal phase. Symptoms can last anywhere from a few days before bleeding or can manifest throughout the last two weeks of the cycle. Symptoms can strike women at any age and resolve at menopause. This is why women like Grace and so many others with PMDD beg their doctors to take their ovaries out. Because without ovaries, there are no cycles. And without cycles there is no suffering. While this solution is drastic, painful, permanent, and replete with the potential for horrible side effects (ranging from the inability to have children to osteoporosis), for women with severe PMDD, it can feel like a small price to pay to feel like themselves again.

DO I HAVE PMDD?

If you have five or more of the following symptoms (and *at least one* has to be related to mood), you may have PMDD.

- **Symptoms:** emotional unsteadiness, irritability/anger, depressed mood, anxiety, tension, loss of interest, difficulty concentrating, fatigue, marked appetite changes, overeating or food cravings, insomnia or hypersomnia (sleepiness), feeling emotionally overwhelmed, and experiencing physical symptoms such as breast tenderness, bloating, or headaches.

- **To meet diagnostic criteria for PMDD, the symptoms must:** (a) significantly impair function, and affect relationships and work or school performance, and (b) must emerge in the luteal phase of the menstrual cycle and get better within a few days of bleeding.

One of the things that can make PMDD tricky to diagnose is the fact that it can look like other things. For example, as we learned in chapter 9, the luteal phase is a time when other conditions can get exacerbated. And this includes the symptoms of things like major depressive disorder, panic disorder, eating disorders, psychotic disorder, and borderline personality disorder. If you're someone who has an existing psychiatric disorder, it can be hard to tell whether you have PMDD or a premenstrual exacerbation (PME) of an existing psychiatric condition. It can be particularly hard to distinguish if the psychiatric condition is something that you can muscle through without clinical intervention. In these cases, what looks like PMDD may just be the magnification of symptoms that tend to lie just beneath the surface in the follicular phase. Sometimes, this distinction doesn't matter that much in terms of treatment, but other times it can.

If you think that you may have PMDD, start tracking your symptoms, using something like the PMDD symptom tracker from the International Association for Premenstrual Disorders (which can be found at https://www.iapmd.org/shop/p/iapmd-pmds-symptom-tracker), and talk to your doctor about your concerns. During your conversation with your doctor, be sure to mention whether you have any personal or current history of psychiatric illness or mood disorders. You might also want to check out some of the other wonderful resources available from IAPMD. They have a self-screening quiz as well as a ton of wonderful well-researched resources to help sufferers.

This chapter will share what we currently know and do not know about PMDD, including the latest research into what causes it, who is vulnerable, and possible treatment options. This will include a discussion of both pharmaceutical (e.g., antidepressants and the birth control pill) and lifestyle-based options aimed at addressing symptoms and improving resilience to hormonal changes.

Although we have a long way to go before there are an acceptable number of treatment options available to help reduce women's PMDD suffering, it is my hope that you will find some new ideas about things that might work for you or someone you love who has this heartbreaking condition.

The Many Causes of PMDD

If you are a woman who has PMDD, research shows that you see the world differently in the luteal phase than the follicular . . . and in ways that are not positive for mental health. For example, women with PMDD have cognitive processing differences that can contribute to anxiety and sensory overload. Women with PMDD startle more easily in the luteal phase and are also less adept at filtering out unnecessary sensory information (called sensorimotor gating) at this time. These differences can contribute to feeling overwhelmed or on edge, as well as experiencing anxiety and heightened sensitivity to sensory stimuli (for example, lights and sounds), in the luteal phase. If you talk to women who have PMDD you'll learn that these feelings are very common. They can become overwhelmed by sounds, lights, and social situations that don't bother them at all in the follicular phase.

Women with PMDD also have a heightened negativity bias when viewing others' faces in the luteal phase than do healthy controls, and, making matters worse, they're less able to regulate their emotional responses to them. This means they're more likely to perceive emotions like anger and hostility in the faces of people making neutral expressions, and less able to control the urge to lash out in response to the feeling that they're being attacked. These patterns are compounded by the fact that PMDD impairs women's cognitive control over their emotions in the luteal phase, which can make it harder for sufferers to talk themselves out of feeling things they don't want to feel. This is why many women with PMDD report getting stuck in cycles of hurt and anger. They can't escape the feeling that they're unloved, which causes them to act out in anger, which then makes them feel like their relationships have been irreparably damaged by their responses, and the cycle continues because they're not able to get their brain unstuck from these negative feedback loops.

Although PMDD often appears and disappears with the arrival and exit of progesterone across the cycle, progesterone levels themselves don't seem to be the culprit behind women's symptoms. Research looking at differences in progesterone levels between those who have and do not have PMDD find no differences in their hormone levels.* Instead, the problem seems to be that women with PMDD are less able to gracefully navigate the huge number of neurobiological changes that occur in response to rapidly changing hormone levels in the luteal phase,† especially those stemming from changes in GABAergic activity in the second half of the cycle.

Here's a brief refresher on those changes in GABAergic activity:

- GABA is the main inhibitory neurotransmitter in our brain. This means that it is the primary mechanism by which our brain sloooowwwws itself down and creates inner calm. It's what we feel when we've had a massage or a martini. Our brain slows and we feel more relaxed.
- One of the most potent stimulators of GABA receptors in the brain is the progesterone metabolite allopregnanolone.

---

* Interestingly, there may be some differences in the severity of mood symptoms among women without PMDD based on differences in progesterone, although different research finds different patterns. In one study, researchers found that mood symptoms were worse in women during ovulatory compared to anovulatory cycles, which would suggest that progesterone makes mood worse. However, in a different study, women were followed over the course of two cycles and it was found that cycles that had lower progesterone levels were those that were associated with worse mood symptoms. Takeaway? There may be a relationship between progesterone levels and mood symptoms among women without PMDD, but we are not yet sure exactly what that relationship is.

† This is also why women who get PMDD tend to have a rougher go with perimenopause and the postpartum period. Both are also periods of huge hormonal change, and women who lack the ability to quickly adjust to rapid hormonal changes tend to suffer the most during these transitions.

This calming neurosteroid gets released when the body breaks down progesterone. When progesterone levels rise, ALLO levels rise. When progesterone levels fall, ALLO levels fall.
- When progesterone and ALLO levels rise, the brain calms down. When progesterone and ALLO levels fall, the brain can feel overwhelmed.

For most of us, the changes in GABAergic activity that occur across the cycle are felt like small waves in an ocean. We feel a little more tired and relaxed when ALLO levels rise, and we feel a little jumpier and more on edge when ALLO levels fall. But we continue to feel more or less like ourselves because our neurons are able to make the necessary adjustments in the availability and function of our GABA receptors to help minimize the impact of these changes on how we feel.

For women with PMDD, these things just don't seem to happen the way they're supposed to. Research suggests that for some women, PMDD symptoms occur in response to their neurotransmitter receptors being less able to make the physiological adjustments to the changes in GABAergic activity that occur in the luteal phase. They feel overwhelmed or underwhelmed by GABAergic activity because their GABA receptors aren't able to keep up. For others, symptoms are created by their bodies being *too* quick to adjust to the changes in GABAergic activity in the luteal phase, creating symptoms of withdrawal. This leads them to feel symptoms of GABA withdrawal (anxiety, psychological distress) even when levels of ALLO are high. Regardless of the process by which it occurs, the inability to adaptively regulate changes in GABAergic activity in the luteal phase can cause symptoms like anxiety, depression, irritability, headaches, low energy, sleep disturbances, and body aches and pain.

But it's not just changes in GABAergic activity that wreak havoc on mood with PMDD. These symptoms can also arise from changes in the activities of the neurotransmitter serotonin, which is also impacted by rapidly changing hormone levels in the luteal phase.

If you need a quick refresher on what serotonin is, it is a neurotransmitter known for making our brains feel good. And, as you might imagine given how terrible most women with PMDD feel, research finds that women who have PMDD have serotonergic activity in the luteal phase that does not look like that of their nonsuffering peers. Compared to healthy controls, women with PMDD have blunted serotonin production (they make less of the neurotransmitter), lower levels of serotonin circulating in whole blood, and fewer serotonin receptors available to pick up the signal. Women with PMDD also exhibit diminished sensitivity to serotonin in the luteal phase than they do in the follicular—which means that their bodies are less responsive to it—which is not a pattern that is observed in healthy controls. And when you look at PMDD symptoms, many of them are things that we tend to see when there are serotonergic shenanigans in the system. Low mood, food cravings, and feeling mentally foggy are all common symptoms of dysregulation in the serotonergic system and also of PMDD.

It seems clear that women with PMDD seem to have dysfunctional neurotransmitter activity in response to the hormonal changes that occur across the cycle. But the thing that is far less clear is *why* this happens in the first place. Why is it that most women are able to gracefully navigate changes in neurotransmission in response to hormonal changes across the cycle, while others are not? And what is it about them that makes their systems acclimate to ALLO too quickly or become less sensitive to serotonin released in the luteal phase? To me, these are the million-dollar questions. Because once you have an explanation for these differences, you could potentially help the body heal PMDD instead of simply treating the symptoms.

Although study of this area is relatively new, there is a small body of research that is beginning to uncover some of the factors that contribute to the lack of resilience to hormonal changes that creates PMDD. This research suggests that chronic stress and inflammation might each play a role in creating a neurobiological landscape that is less able to keep one's mood stable when the seas of hormonal change begin rocking the boat.

The Why Behind the How: Stress and Inflammation in PMDD

The ability to ride lightly on the waves of hormonal change requires a lot of physiological dexterity. The brain and body have to be able to quickly adjust to the huge number of biological changes in response to rapidly rising and falling levels of sex hormones. When our bodies are able to do this effectively, our hormonal changes across the cycle are often felt like small(ish) shifts in our internal topography. We can feel ourselves crest a hill or descend from a peak, but it happens slowly and without the risk of altitude sickness. This is what changes in our cycle are supposed to feel like.

When things don't feel this way, and our changing hormonal landscape feels more like we're driving off a cliff than coasting down a mesa, it means our body's ability to adapt to hormonal change has been compromised. This often means that there is a problem with our stress response, the system in our body that is responsible for allowing us to adapt to changing physical, physiological, and social environments. Whether we are experiencing changes in temperature, threat levels, or something else in our internal or external environment, our stress response allows our body to deal with the temporary upheaval and get things back to some semblance of a physiological status quo.

Given the important role that the stress response plays in our body's ability to navigate physiological change, researchers suspect that it may also play an important role in our ability to navigate hormonal changes. Because our sex hormones create physiological changes in our bodies from head to toe, having a high-functioning stress response might be the key to navigating these changes without feeling too much upheaval. When the stress response system is working well, we should expect to see more mood stability and fewer menstrual-related symptoms. And when it is not working well, we should see dysregulation and mood-related symptoms like those we see in women with PMS and PMDD.

Although this is a relatively new idea, there's a growing body of research that supports the theory. Much research finds, for example, that having a history of trauma or chronic stress exposure—both of which are known to cause dysregulation of the stress response—are strong risk factors for the development of PMDD. In one cross-sectional study of nearly four thousand women, researchers found that trauma history significantly increased women's risk of subsequently being diagnosed with PMDD. And this relationship was found to hold after controlling for a number of factors that could have alternatively accounted for this greater risk (for example, differences in socioeconomic status). Similar results have been found in case-control and longitudinal studies. Researchers in one study found that women with PMDD were 6.7 times more likely to report childhood sexual abuse than controls. And a separate longitudinal study of more than three thousand women found that those who had experienced physical and emotional abuse in childhood were 2.1 and 2.6 times, respectively, more likely to have PMS or PMDD as adults than women without such a history.

The primary cause of this heightened PMDD risk profile for women who have suffered trauma is believed to be dysregulation of the hypothalamic-pituitary-adrenal (HPA)* axis, which is the arm of the stress response responsible for releasing the stress hormone cortisol. Although cortisol is often treated as a physiological boogeyman (because too much of it can wreak total havoc on all the body's systems), it is actually an important part of how our body is able to respond to and recover from stress. It creates a number of physio-

---

* HPA axis = hypothalamic-pituitary-adrenal axis, which is the communication pathway between your brain (specifically, the hypothalamus), the pituitary gland (the little pea-size gland at the base of your brain that directs traffic with all your hormone-releasing organs), and your adrenal glands (the little blobs on the top of your kidneys that release the stress hormone cortisol). This pathway is responsible for regulating the cortisol-release part of our stress response. The other half (in case you're interested . . . and even if you're not) is the sympathetic stress response, which is responsible for the fight-or-flight portion of our stress response. This is coordinated by the hormone epinephrine, which is also released by your adrenals.

logical changes that allow us to cope with, learn from, and adapt to stress. Having a high-functioning HPA axis is necessary for our bodies to navigate various forms of stress, including our changing sex hormones across the cycle.

Unfortunately, research suggests that the HPA axes of women with PMDD might not work the way they're supposed to. Compared to healthy controls, women with PMDD have higher morning cortisol in the luteal phase and, throughout the cycle, have lower evening cortisol, a later daily cortisol peak, a delayed cortisol awakening response, and a lower cortisol response to stress than what is observed in healthy controls. These are the sort of patterns that we tend to see in people with PTSD and severe depression, suggesting that those with PMDD might not be able to cope with stress as well as healthy controls.

Alterations in the HPA axis, like those observed in women with PMDD, can also create higher-than-normal levels of inflammation, which is also known to diminish hormonal resilience and contribute to poor mental health. Researchers have long noted a link between inflammatory activity and problems with mental health and psychopathology, making it a possible contributor to PMDD mood changes. Although there is a long way to go before we know what, if any, role inflammation plays in PMDD symptoms, there is some research linking elevated levels of inflammation to negative mood symptoms across the cycle. This research—particularly when it is considered alongside the mounting evidence that inflammation is one of the key culprits behind poor mental health—suggests that inflammatory activity may be an important player in the development of PMDD and the lack of general resilience to hormonal changes.

Lastly, researchers have identified some genetic risk factors that can decrease women's resilience to hormonal changes across the cycle. It suggests that women with PMDD may have an inherited vulnerability to hormonal fluctuations. While no single "PMDD gene" has been identified (genes don't work that way), studies suggest that certain polymorphisms in genes related to serotonin regulation, such as the SLC6A4 gene, may impact women's risk of PMDD. Variants of this gene can affect serotonin reuptake, potentially leading to altered mood regulation during the luteal phase. Additionally, genes involved in the function of the HPA axis and hormone receptors, particularly the progesterone receptor gene (PGR), may also influence how the body responds to hormonal changes. This genetic sensitivity to hormone fluctuations can result in the mood disturbances and physical symptoms that define PMDD, making this an important area for future research.

Although research is still a long way from being able to identify all the causes of PMDD (and I say causes with an *s* because it seems pretty clear that the path to PMDD is likely multicausal), I am hopeful about the future. In the meantime, there are a growing number of options for women seeking relief. We will turn to those now.

Let's talk about these options, starting with the traditional medical approach of prescription drugs and then following with a discussion of nonprescription options. I'm presenting both of these approaches to you because different women find different strategies most beneficial. I'm hoping that this will give you the information you need to begin conversations with your health-care provider about which approach might work best for you.

This Is Your PMDD on Drugs

If you have gone to your doctor for PMDD, chances are you were offered selective serotonin reuptake inhibitors (SSRIs) as the first line of defense in treating your symptoms. They're currently considered the gold-standard treatment for PMDD by the American College of Obstetricians and Gynecologists, making them a treatment of choice for many of those who write prescriptions. While it's highly unlikely that PMDD is ultimately caused by a Prozac deficiency, research finds that SSRIs like Prozac do seem to help many women feel better. For example, studies comparing symptoms of women taking SSRIs for three months to untreated women or women taking a placebo find a 50 percent decrease in luteal-phase mood symptoms among those being treated compared to those who are not. And recent meta-analyses looking at the effectiveness of multiple types of SSRI treatments[*] across several different studies find the same thing. Women assigned to take SSRIs for PMDD have better symptom improvement than those on placebos, suggesting that SSRIs can be an important tool in some women's war against PMDD.

The unfortunate thing about SSRI treatment is that many women don't want to take them. And this is understandable. They mess with neurotransmitters, which means they mess with the brain (which is something we should always be incredibly cautious with). And they often come with a number of undesirable side effects that can make for a not-great user experience. They can include things like nausea, insomnia, headaches, and loss of sexual desire and function (which doesn't always go away when SSRI use is discontinued).[†]

The good news for women who are open to using SSRIs to treat PMDD is that research suggests that they can be used effectively to treat PMDD without the need to be taken every day. That is, women can minimize their exposure to negative side effects while still getting the mood-balancing effects of the drugs by taking SSRIs only when they're feeling bad. Because unlike what is required for SSRIs to be effective at treating depression (continuous use for several weeks), SSRI therapy for PMDD can begin working within *hours* and only needs to be taken when women are symptomatic (in the luteal phase). And this is a BFD[‡] because it means less drug exposure, fewer unpleasant side effects, and more patient control if and when the medication is taken.

The reason that SSRIs can be dosed intermittently for PMDD but not depression is because the mechanism by which they improve

---

[*] In case you were wondering, the SSRIs studied were citalopram, escitalopram, fluoxetine, fluvoxamine, paroxetine, sertraline, or zimelidine. They have also looked at venlafaxine and duloxetine, which are not SSRIs but have a similar mechanism of action at low doses.

[†] Yes, post-SSRI sexual dysfunction is a thing. And it is common enough to have been given its own charming acronym: PSSD.

[‡] Big f*cking deal.

symptoms differs for each condition. Although in both treatment contexts SSRIs work by increasing the availability of serotonin in the synaptic cleft, it is what this extra serotonin does to help you feel better that differs depending on what ails you. In the case of depression, this surfeit of serotonin is believed to change one's mood by initiating structural and functional changes in the brain that increase neuroplasticity and improve serotonergic function (which is why it takes so darn long to feel better—brain changes take time). In the case of PMDD, though, this extra serotonin is believed to improve mood by increasing the rate by which progesterone is converted into mood-stabilizing neurosteroids like ALLO. This helps keep ALLO levels high and steady, taking the edge off the emotional roller coaster that can result from the rapid rise and fall of progesterone. Because this action doesn't require changes in the brain that can take several weeks to unfold, the mood improvement effects are felt almost immediately upon use.

The following SSRI drugs have been tested and found effective for symptom relief using a flexible dosing regimen (i.e., a regimen that allows women to take the drugs only when symptomatic): citalopram, escitalopram, fluoxetine, paroxetine, and sertraline. By the time this book is in your hands, there may be other drugs that have been found to work well in this sort of dosing context. It's important to note that research finds that not all PMDD symptoms respond equally to flexible versus continuous dosing. For example, flexible dosing is particularly useful for treating symptoms related to irritability and mood swings; however, it may be less effective than continuous dosing for treating depressed mood and somatic symptoms like headaches and fatigue. So if you are considering SSRI treatment, you will want to spend some time talking with your doctor about the specifics of your symptoms and your side effect concerns to determine which product and dosing option might work best for you and your needs.

Although SSRIs are currently the go-to treatment of many prescribers, they don't work for everyone. Somewhere between 12 and 50 percent of women who try SSRIs for PMDD will be nonresponders. This is important to know at the outset since there is a chance that you will need to come up with a plan B for treatment. One potential option is a newer class of antidepressant drugs called SNRIs (serotonin-norepinephrine reuptake inhibitors) that are showing early success as treatments for PMDD (although, as of this writing, it is unclear whether these newer drugs are effective for women who don't respond to SSRIs). Another option for women who are open to treating their PMDD pharmacologically but do not respond to SSRI treatment is a medication called dutasteride. Like SSRIs, dutasteride acts on processes related to women's changing levels of ALLO in the luteal phase. However, with dutasteride, instead of stabilizing mood by keeping ALLO levels *high*, it stabilizes mood by keeping ALLO levels *low*. It does this by blocking the actions of 5-alpha-reductase (an enzyme produced in the body that—in addition to converting testosterone into its most potent form—prevents conversion of progesterone to allopregnanolone). By keeping levels of ALLO low and steady, dutasteride is able to prevent the volatility in levels of this calming neurosteroid that tend to occur when levels of progesterone are rapidly changing. Research finds that dutasteride decreases a range of PMDD symptoms, including irritability, anxiety, sadness, food cravings, and bloating. And the best part is it seems to do this while producing only minimal side effects. For these reasons, dutasteride is an off-label option[*] that some doctors are offering patients who experience intolerable side effects or do not benefit from treatment with SSRIs.

The other prescription option to alleviate symptoms of PMDD is the birth control pill. While SSRIs work by smoothing out levels of ALLO to minimize psychological turbulence, the pill works by flattening women's hormonal changes across the cycle, which keeps levels of hormonally sensitive neurotransmission constant.

When women are on hormonal birth control, the synthetic progesterone (progestins) in the treatment gets picked up by progesterone receptors in the brain. When progesterone receptors are activated, it makes the brain believe that ovulation has occurred and pregnancy

---

[*] No joke: this stuff is usually prescribed to treat enlarged prostates.

could be imminent. Because the body doesn't want to ovulate again before it knows for certain that it's not pregnant already (serial pregnancies would be physiologically disastrous), the brain tells the ovaries to hold off on stimulating new egg follicles until progesterone stops being released. This means that eggs won't ever develop, ovulation won't occur, and hormones won't be produced—and hormones won't rise and fall in ways that can produce rapid changes in neurotransmission that create PMDD symptoms.

Although shutting down ovulation and hormone production by delivering a daily dose of synthetic hormones can make some women feel pretty awful, research finds it to be hugely palliative to women with PMDD. Because if you're someone who feels bad in response to hormonal changes, taking something that shuts down those changes and replaces them with a consistent dose of a synthetic can make you feel a whole lot better than how you feel when you're cycling. The research evidence is particularly strong for combined oral contraceptives containing the progestin drospirenone (3 milligrams) plus ethinyl estradiol (20 µg). A number of randomized, double-blind placebo-controlled trials—the gold standard—have found that these treatments improve mood in women with PMDD relative to the placebo group. There is also good research support for continuous dosing of hormonal contraceptives containing the progestin levonorgestrel (90 micrograms) and ethinyl estradiol (20 micrograms). These are the types of birth control pills that you take for several months in a row without taking placebo pills that give you a withdrawal bleed (or what looks like a period).* This one can be particularly helpful to

---

* No, the "period" you get when you're taking hormonal birth control isn't actually a period. It is triggered by the drop in hormones that occurs in response to switching from the pills in your pill pack that contain hormones to the sugar pills that do not contain hormones. Although this is similar to what happens when you get your period (periods are also caused by a drop in hormones), it's not really a period since you aren't shedding an endometrial lining. You don't build up much of an endometrial lining when you are on hormonal birth control because of the hormonal profile of these drugs. This is also why hormonal birth control can be helpful to women with endometriosis (it prevents overproliferation of cells in the endome-

women sensitive to hormonal changes since it minimizes the number of hormonal peaks and valleys women experience each year by minimizing the number of times women transition to placebo pills.

Hormonal birth control, though, can come with a number of side effects (I write about these extensively in *This Is Your Brain on Birth Control*, so I won't repeat all that information here). It's important to consider your tolerance for these side effects when making a decision about whether this treatment is right for you. It's also worth noting that research finds that some types of hormonal birth control can make women's PMDD *worse*. For example, progestin-only methods like the progestin-only pill (this is the one you can now get over the counter), the hormonal IUD (which contains the progestin levonorgestrel), the birth control implant (which contains the progestin etonogestrel), or the birth control shot (which contains the progestin medroxyprogesterone) are often found to make the symptoms of PMDD and other mood disorders worse. So you need to make sure you are working with a doctor who has some background in treating PMDD with hormonal birth control to make sure that all the risks and benefits of different types of treatments are taken into account.

In addition to SSRIs and hormonal birth control, there are also a handful of other interventions available for women with PMDD that work by either directly or indirectly affecting the hormonal changes across the cycle that are believed to create PMDD symptoms. For example, some treatments work by blocking progesterone receptors so it's never "read" by the body. There are also treatments that work by blocking or preventing the release of gonadotropin-releasing hormone (GnRH, which shuts down ovulation by preventing the brain from telling the pituitary to stimulate the ovaries to begin egg development). These sorts of treatments are relatively new, the results on their effectiveness are mixed, and they tend to be used only in women

---

trium), and why it is safe to take for several months in a row without having a withdrawal bleed. If you aren't proliferating a lot of endometrial cells (and women on the pill are not), there is a much lower probability that you will have wonky cells hanging around that could develop into cancer or create other problems.

who have failed to find relief from more conventional treatments. This is particularly true for those hormones blocking GnRH, since it suppresses women's own hormone production and doesn't replace them with synthetics, creating a hormonal state that is comparable to menopause. When experienced too early, this can cause issues with bone density, cardiovascular health, brain health, and a whole bunch of other issues that tend to pop up when your levels of sex hormones are much lower than what they should be for a woman of reproductive age.

Although drug-based therapies aren't for everyone (and women are growing increasingly wary of drug-based therapies being the only options offered to them by their physicians), there are a lot of women who find them helpful and even lifesaving. If you think you might be one of these women, I hope the information provided here will give you a place to start in conversations with your doctor about treatment. Research estimates that women with PMDD often take years to find a correct diagnosis and even longer to get in touch with the right treatment. And since the right treatment can—for some women—literally mean the difference between life and death, time is of the essence. It is my wish that this information helps you get the treatment you want sooner than later, regardless of what that treatment looks like for you.

Soothing Your Cycle Drug-Free

Although you may have been told that treating PMDD will require the use of prescription drugs, this simply isn't true. There are a number of ways you can support your body and decrease symptoms naturally using your body's own capacity for healing and the support of a well-trained therapist. Some of them are aimed at improving the health of your body (healthy bodies are better able to recover from stress and have more neuroplasticity than unhealthy bodies). And some are aimed at taking a more targeted approach to managing symptoms through the use of psychotherapy, exercise, dietary changes, or supplements. Although this section is shorter than the section dedicated to explaining the use of prescription drugs, don't take this as an indication that prescription drugs are the only answer. They're not. There is just more research being done on drug-based therapies for PMDD than there is for some of the nondrug-based treatments.

First and most importantly, if you have PMDD, I highly encourage you to take steps to help support the health of your body, because being in good health can make the difference between tolerable and intolerable PMDD symptoms. Although it is unlikely that adopting a healthier lifestyle is going to solve all of your problems (PMDD is often more powerful than a good night of sleep and a five-mile run), it can take the edge off symptoms and help complement whatever other treatments you pursue in the name of feeling better. Bodies that are well nourished, well rested, and exercised have lower inflammation and are more resilient to stress than bodies that are poorly nourished, poorly rested, and sedentary. This means that anything you can do to help promote the health of your body (which also means the health of your brain!) is going to increase your resilience to the physiological and emotional shake-ups that happen in the luteal phase. Getting enough sleep, eating a diet made up primarily of whole, unprocessed foods, getting sunlight* (or using a UV lamp that mimics the effects of sunlight), and getting regular physical activity will put you in a much better position to feel better in the luteal phase than you would be if you weren't being mindful of your health.

I recognize that taking care of your body can be a whole lot easier said than done (this is especially true if you are in the throes of a depressive episode), but even small steps can help. You don't need to turn your life totally upside down to start nudging your body in the

---

* Sunlight exposure is good for us in a lot of different ways. Research finds that sunlight exposure has tremendous mental health benefits: It allows our bodies to synthesize vitamin D (critical for physical and mental health), and if we view it first thing in the morning when the sun is still rising, it helps us set our circadian clocks. Obviously, you don't want to overdo it so that your risk of skin cancer increases, but sunlight exposure can be an important tool in your mental health tool kit.

direction of better health and greater hormonal resilience. Consider having your morning coffee outside to get some direct sunlight exposure (good for synthesizing mood-boosting vitamin D and getting your circadian clock set for a better night of sleep). If you drive to work or school, park a block or two away from where you need to be so that you can stretch your legs a bit before you have to sit at your desk or drive home at night. Find a couple of healthy recipes that look tasty and cook them.* The thing I love about preparing healthy food is that it nourishes your body and it gets you moving (I get an extra three to four thousand steps clocked on days that I spend an hour or so cooking dinner than I do on days when I don't). It's a win-win.

Any steps you take to improve the quality of your health—even small ones—will help in your fight against PMDD. They will also promote healthy cycles and hormone production, which make for a healthier, more balanced you. I will spend more time talking about specific steps that all women can take to improve health and hormonal resilience in the next chapter. For now, consider taking an audit of things in your life that you are willing to adjust to make room for better health.

In addition to doing things to help support the health of your body, research also finds that there are some targeted nonmedical interventions that can lead to significant improvements in women's PMDD treatments. They include cognitive behavioral therapy (CBT), the use of supplements, and the use of physical activity and exercise. We will start by talking about CBT since it is the nonpharmaceutical intervention that seems to have the best success rates.

If you've never heard of CBT, it's a form of psychotherapy that works by helping people identify negative thought patterns that can make them feel bad, challenging the assumptions behind the

---

* If you are new to healthy cooking, start with simple recipes that don't have too many ingredients or steps. It is easy to get overwhelmed when you're first learning your way around the kitchen. Also, remember to prep/measure all the ingredients before you start the actual cooking so that everything is ready for you when you need it.

thought patterns, and then helping replace them with more positive and realistic ways of thinking. For example, if PMDD makes you feel sad and anxious because you feel like everyone hates you, your therapist will first work with you to help identify the ways of thinking that are making you feel bad (here: thinking everyone hates you). Then, your therapist will help you challenge those thoughts and assumptions in ways that make you think beyond your current perception (e.g., "Is it possible that everyone might not hate you?") and help you reframe your perceptions of reality in a way that allows you to cope with them differently. Although the specifics of how CBT is practiced can vary from therapist to therapist (which is why it's a good idea to try a couple of different therapists before deciding whether it may or may not work for you), it generally works by reshaping responses to negative mood-triggering events or people and helping patients develop coping strategies for negative patterns of thinking and feeling.

A pretty significant body of research finds that CBT can help alleviate women's PMDD mood symptoms. Experimental research regularly finds that women who undergo CBT treatments have significant symptom improvement compared to women in a control group (women who are not given CBT treatment). Systematic reviews of research looking at the relative effectiveness of CBT versus SSRI treatments—which are currently considered the gold standard—find similarly positive effects on women's symptoms for both types of treatments (although SSRIs have a slight leg up on treating anxiety symptoms), which is wonderful news for women seeking to avoid medication. Better yet, new research using internet-based cognitive-behavioral therapy—which makes treatment less of a hassle and time commitment—shows similar results to in-person appointments. This makes this form of treatment more accessible to a broader range of women than ever before since not everyone has the type of flexible schedule that allows for in-person therapy appointments. Although there is a still a lot of research that needs to be done before we know who will and won't be helped by CBT treatment for PMDD (much

COMPLEMENTARY AND ALTERNATIVE ORAL MEDICATION DOSING FOR TREATMENT OF PMS OR PMDD

TREATMENT	DOSE
Vitex agnus-castus	8 mg to 41 mg daily
Kami-shoyo-san	2.5 g three times per day
Saffron	15 mg twice daily
Hypericum perforatum	600 mg daily
Chamomile	100 mg to 400 mg daily
Vitamin B_6 (pyridoxine)	50 mg to 100 mg daily[a]
Vitamin B_1 (thiamine)	100 mg daily
Vitamin D	*[b]
Calcium	500 mg to 1,200 mg daily
Zinc (elemental)	30 mg to 50 mg daily
Magnesium	250 mg daily
Omega-3 fatty acids	500 mg to 2000 mg daily[c]
Myo-inositol	0.6 mg in gel capsule or 2 g in powder

[a] *Higher doses tested, but upper limit of 100 mg per day recommended for adults.*
[b] *Dose suggestion cannot be determined per available evidence.*
[c] *Variable DHA and EPA composition.*

of the research in this area has been done on relatively small samples of women with a broad range of symptoms and illness severity), it might be worth considering.

In addition to CBT, there is also some research supporting the use of vitamins/supplements and exercise as treatments for PMDD. Although these sorts of treatments are often recommended for PMS more than they are PMDD (especially more serious forms of PMDD), they may offer symptom relief to some women, making them worth a mention.

First, let's talk supplements. Above is a list of treatments that have received some empirical support as being helpful to women with PMDD (we're defining helpful as something that has been found to decrease PMS or PMDD symptoms in at least one reasonably well-designed study).* Next to the type of treatment is the dosing that has been found to be effective at improving symptoms. You can learn more about each of these treatments using the references I have cited in the notes at the back of the book. You can also learn more about them in chapter 6, on mood. At the end of that chapter, I spend a lot of time talking about ways to increase intake of vitamins and minerals known to support mood in the luteal phase, using either supplements or food-based sources. Consider using the resources in this book as a starting point for a conversation with your care provider about possible treatments that might work for you. He or she will be able to weigh in on how advisable or inadvisable a given supplement might be for you and your symptoms, given your personal health history and other considerations that could affect how it makes you feel.

There is also a fairly impressive body of research supporting the use of exercise as a treatment for PMDD mood symptoms. This is something I love because most of us can do this without having to spend any of our hard-earned cash. Whether it's swimming, Pilates, yoga, or even something as simple as walking or dancing in your living room, research finds that women assigned to an exercise treatment (where they're told to exercise regularly for a period of time, usually for eight weeks or more) have fewer PMDD mood symptoms than women experimentally assigned to a control condition. These results are echoed in a recent (2020) meta-analysis looking at the effectiveness of exercise as a treatment for premenstrual mood symptoms.† The conclusion of this research was that exercise produces

---

* At least in some studies. Note that many of the studies looking at nontraditional therapies tend to have relatively small samples and often have conflicting results. Nonetheless, each of these interventions has some research support, but none of them is likely to be a magic bullet that makes everything better.

† Note that these were generally studies conducted on women with PMS, not PMDD. Although there is a reason to assume that interventions that improve PMS mood symptoms should also improve PMDD mood symptoms (they should if the mechanisms that cause the symptoms are the same, which they seem to be), we cannot be certain of this.

significant improvements in the mood relative to what is observed in women who don't exercise.

Although the exact mechanisms by which changes in diet, use of supplements, and exercise decrease PMDD symptoms are unknown, it's likely that these interventions work along several pathways. In particular, they likely help decrease inflammation (good for mental health and neuroplasticity), improve neurotransmission by improving the health of the brain, and (with exercise) increase the functioning of the stress response. Although there is still a lot to be learned about the role of nutrition, supplements, and exercise on the health of the brain and our resilience to hormonal changes, many women find that making these changes can be helpful in minimizing symptoms, and you might too.

Lastly, I want to mention one other area that my research lab is currently investigating as being potentially therapeutic in the treatment of PMDD, and that is stimulation of the vagus nerve. The vagus nerve is a gigantic bundle of nerve fibers that extends down from the brain and branches out into the periphery of the body to provide the brain with information about how all of our different parts are doing. It also helps regulate our autonomic nervous system (which is the part of the nervous system that shifts us from fight-or-flight into rest-and-digest mode).

Recently, researchers have taken to stimulating the vagus nerve to help improve symptoms of issues stemming from stress dysregulation. Vagus nerve stimulation (VNS) entails delivering mild electrical impulses to the nerve, either through a small, implanted device or (like we do in my lab) in a noninvasive way by delivering impulses to the tragus on your ear (that little cartilage triangle next to your ear canal that is closest to your jawbone). These impulses activate the nerve, promoting a calming "rest-and-digest" response, which can help reduce stress, inflammation, and symptoms of conditions like depression, epilepsy, and even migraine. By improving vagal tone—the nerve's ability to perform efficiently—VNS has shown potential to balance the nervous system and enhance overall physical and mental well-being.

VNS has been found to be effective at treating depression, anxiety, and—because of its therapeutic effects on inflammation—endometriosis (painful overgrowth of the endometrial lining). Given the successes and the shared mechanisms involved in each of these conditions and PMDD, my graduate student Savannah Hastings has begun to explore the possibility of noninvasive VNS on PMDD symptoms. It is my hope that by the time you are reading this book we have begun to see this as a possible treatment option for women looking to manage their PMDD without the use of medication.

I will close this section by adding that one last-ditch intervention that women sometimes pursue to eliminate PMDD is a surgical hysterectomy with a bilaterial ovary removal. This is a treatment option that works (removing the source of progesterone production will do that for a person), but I wouldn't recommend it. It should only be used as a last-line treatment because it is so barbaric and has a number of downstream health consequences. Because ovary removal is something that removes the organ responsible for most of your sex hormone production, having this surgery will put you into early menopause. Because there are a number of health issues that crop up for women who go through early menopause that most of us should try to avoid (e.g., a heightened risk of osteoporosis and dementia), this is something that should only be considered by women for whom there simply are no other solutions.

Things You Can Do Today to Help Manage Your PMDD

If you think you may have PMDD, let me start by saying how sorry I am that you were dealt this hand. As someone who has been in the women's health space for some time now, I have met so many who struggle with PMDD, and their stories are heartbreaking. Many feel like they have spent half of their adult lives at war with themselves. And most of them have had a long, painful path to get from symptoms to diagnosis (and then from diagnosis to treatment). Thankfully, there are some things that you can do today to help speed things along if you hope to seek a diagnosis. And there are also things you can do to help make your symptoms feel more tolerable and manageable:

- If you think you have PMDD, make an appointment with your doctor to talk about your symptoms and get a diagnosis. Even if you plan to try to tackle your symptoms with lifestyle-based modifications rather than prescription drugs, having a diagnosis can help you understand what is actually going on with your body and help rule out the possibility that your symptoms are the result of something else altogether (for example, a PME of an existing psychiatric condition, seasonal affective disorder, or something like hypothyroidism or a vitamin D deficiency). Find a healthcare provider you trust and make an appointment to get the ball rolling on a diagnosis. Your care provider can also be an excellent resource for strategizing a treatment plan, whether that means using prescription drugs, finding a recommended CBT therapist, or trying a lifestyle-based intervention.
- Start tracking your symptoms today. And make sure you date your entries as soon as you begin tracking. Any doctor you see for your PMDD symptoms is going to ask you to track your cycle for at least two months before they will give you a diagnosis. Although this can feel really annoying when you're waiting to get a diagnosis, it helps your doctor make sure that your symptoms are the result of PMDD and not something else. You can get a head start on this two-month tracking period by beginning now. You can find a wonderful, totally free PMDD cycle-tracking calendar on the IAPMD* website (https://www.iapmd.org

---

* IAPMD is the International Association for Premenstrual Disorders, which is an absolutely wonderful organization that is full of resources for women struggling

/shop/p/iapmd-pmds-symptom-tracker). When you track your symptoms, you want to make note of both their presence (do I have this symptom or not?) and their severity (how bad is it?). Bring your completed tracking calendar to your doctor appointment to see if it can help get you more quickly to a diagnosis and a care strategy that works for you.

- If you are considering cognitive behavioral therapy to help with your PMDD, start researching therapists. Don't simply make an appointment with the first person whose name you see on your Google search. Interview them. Ask to schedule a phone call before your first appointment and ask questions about their approach to CBT, what you can expect in your sessions, and how they benchmark the success of their patients. Asking questions like this will give you an opportunity to see what sort of rapport you have with your potential therapist-to-be and how comfortable they make you feel. Then you can make an appointment with the one (or ones) you think will be the best fit. If after a couple of appointments you're not vibing with your therapist, don't be afraid to try someone else. Sometimes it can take a couple of misses before we find the right fit. Be patient. The results of therapy, when done right, can be so, so worth it. If you don't know where to start in your quest for a therapist who does CBT, *Psychology Today* has a directory of mental health professionals that you can search according to your location and desired specialization (someone who does CBT). If you have health insurance, you can also consult with its care directory if you would like to use someone in network.
- I owe this next beautiful and loving set of self-care instructions to my dear friend Wendy, who told me to do this ex-

---

with premenstrual disorders, including PMDD.

act thing when I was in the midst of a really terrible time in my life. And there are few people I know who could use this loving guidance more than women with PMDD. So here it is: Take immaculate care of yourself. This includes taking care of your physical health—trying to incorporate more movement, sunlight, health-promoting foods, and rest—as well as your mental and spiritual health. Make time for walks in nature, visiting friends and family, and doing other things that make you feel alive and spiritually nourished. Having a healthy body and spirit will allow you to better navigate the physical and psychological upheaval that occurs when our hormones rise and fall dramatically in the luteal phase. It will help increase the odds of success with whichever intervention path you choose to follow.

- Lastly, if you are somebody who is experiencing suicidal ideation as part of your PMDD symptoms (which many women do), please, *please* seek professional help. Call the Suicide and Crisis Lifeline at 988 if you need someone to talk to and do not try to manage your symptoms on your own. I have heard from women who, despite having suicidal thoughts as part of their PMDD experience, were nonetheless afraid to seek treatment because (a) they were afraid of what others would think if they knew how bad things were, or (b) they were afraid to take hormonal birth control or antidepressants to treat their symptoms (even if only temporarily to get them back on their feet) because they were worried about the side effects. If this describes you, please know that while your concerns are valid, they are not worth risking your life for. Please talk to a trusted doctor, psychiatrist, or loved one about how you are feeling so you can start getting the treatment you need. And if a trusted medical professional suggests that you might need medication to help get you in a better place, try to be open to at least considering this as a possibility. Although I am generally of the belief that prescription drugs are overprescribed (because, you know, they are), I recognize the huge value they can provide to those who are suffering. And research suggests that they really can help. Sometimes, going on medication is the right answer. And if you are questioning whether life is worth living because of your PMDD, there's a possibility it may be the right answer for you.

PART III

THE FUTURE IS FEMALE AND HORMONAL

Welcome to the Revolution

CHAPTER 11

RECLAIMING YOUR LUTEAL PHASE

How to promote hormonal balance

When we began this book, we talked about the fact that there are a lot of us who feel like sh*t in the week or two before our periods start. And that a lot of these sh*t-feeling experiences are the result of functional changes going on in our bodies that have become dysfunctional because they've been ignored and we've been following a one-size-fits-all set of rules that are incomplete or based on men. The luteal phase is far more unpleasant for a lot of us than it needs to be, because trying to jam square pegs into round holes rarely works . . . and when it does, it usually causes splinters.

But this isn't the only thing that is contributing to the fact that so many of us feel like sh*t. Because even when we are doing everything right in terms of things like honoring the fact that our fear response and sexual desire can change across the cycle, and making sure that we're feeding ourselves well and exercising in ways that respect our bodies' needs, a lot of us still feel worse than we need to. This is because a lot of the changes we've made to our environments—things like the introduction of processed foods, chronic stress, sedentary lifestyles, and exposure to a host of synthetic chemicals that our ancestors never encountered—have changed our hormonal health for the worse. We are undernourished, and we have too much inflammation, too much stress, and too little social support, which can suppress ovulation and degrade our resilience to hormonal changes. This can make our hormones out of balance and make us less able to roll with the hormonal punches each month.

We're going to spend this chapter talking about how to right these wrongs, and what science has to say about things we can do to improve our hormonal health and resilience. This will start with a discussion about how to support hormonal balance and resilience. As you'll see, there is no reason any of us needs to feel awful in the luteal phase, and most of us can have healthy, balanced cycles most of the time. Next, we will go over how to tell whether you're ovulating (spoiler alert: just because you have regular periods doesn't mean you're ovulating all the time), so that you can keep track of your own hormonal health and balance. Let's dive into the science of how our bodies work to have a better month, every month.

SO WHY DO WE GET PERIOD CRAMPS?

While this isn't exactly a book about periods, I wanted to say a few words about cramps since they're something that a lot of women struggle with at various times of the month.

There are two main types of cramps associated with a typical cycle. There are menstrual cramps, which happen when we're bleeding. These are the result of the uterus contracting to shed its lining. These contractions are triggered by prostaglandins, which are hormonelike substances that promote inflammation and pain, especially when their levels are high. These prostaglandins are also responsible for making us have to poop more (maybe TMI, but them's the facts). A lot of women also get mid-cycle ovulation cramps, also known as mittelschmerz (literally the ugliest word ever, it stems from the German for "middle pain"). These happen when the ovary releases an egg. This can irritate the ovary and surrounding tissues, leading to cramping or a dull ache in one side or throughout your abdomen. Both types of cramps are natural processes, but the severity can vary depending on factors like hormonal balance, diet, and overall health.

Looking to feel better? Of course you are. Here is what my physician friends recommend for improving cramping:

- **Take magnesium.** Magnesium helps relax muscles and reduce inflammation, which can ease cramps. Aim for 300–400 milligrams daily from food (like nuts, seeds, and leafy greens) or supplements.

- **Apply heat.** A heating pad or hot-water bottle can improve blood flow and relax the muscles, providing relief from cramping.

- **Stay hydrated.** Drinking plenty of water can reduce bloating and make cramps less severe.

- **Prioritize anti-inflammatory foods.** Include omega-3-rich foods (like salmon and flaxseeds) and avoid excess sugar and processed foods to lower inflammation.

- **Try herbal teas.** Chamomile, ginger, or peppermint tea may have muscle-relaxing and anti-inflammatory effects. I like peppermint because it also helps me with any type of stomachache, including the ones I get at ovulation.

- **Exercise regularly.** Exercising throughout the cycle makes cramps less severe. And during bleeding, gentle movement, like yoga or walking, can improve circulation and reduce pain.

- **Talk to a doctor.** If cramps are severe or disrupt your life, consult your health-care provider to rule out conditions like endometriosis or fibroids. These issues are super common and make cramping much worse. You shouldn't be in excruciating pain during your period.

Ovulation Suppression and Hormonal Imbalance

Although the idea of hormonal balance and imbalance can sound a little like woo-woo, pseudoscientific wellness-culture speak, there is really nothing woo-woo about it. Hormones get unbalanced when women don't ovulate, because ovulation is the way women's bodies produce most of their progesterone. Although successful ovulation is also responsible for some of our estrogen production, women often continue to release near-ovulatory levels of estrogen during nonovulatory cycles. So, when women don't ovulate, they become estrogen dominant.

Now, you might be tempted to think that an estrogen-only cycle would feel like a sexy twenty-eight-day party with infinite champagne and no chaperones to tell everyone to put their clothes back on, but it usually makes us feel awful. This is because estrogen, while it feels really amazing in short bursts like we experience near ovulation, can quickly become too much if it runs unopposed by progesterone for too long. It can ruin our moods by making us feel irritable, anxious, and depressed. It can increase our risk of fibroids and endometriosis by allowing excessive endometrial proliferation. It can cause migraines by keeping our brain stuck in a highly excitable state. And it can cause pain and fibrocystic changes in the breast by causing runaway proliferation of breast tissue. It's like having a third or fourth day in Las Vegas. You're exhausted, your nerves are shot, and you're like, *Okay, that's enough already*.

Even though you might not suspect that you are someone who frequently experiences hormonal imbalances caused by failure to ovulate, there is a good chance that this has happened to you more frequently than you'd have guessed. This type of hormonal imbalance is incredibly common. Population-based studies of healthy women with regular cycles generally find evidence of ovulation suppression—which is what we call it when a typically ovulating woman experiences ovulatory failure in a given cycle—in about 24 to 37 percent of cycles. If this seems high to you, it's because it is. It seemed high to me too. In fact, for a long time I was convinced that we were doing something wrong in my research lab when studying ovulation because I couldn't believe that many healthy women would experience ovulation suppression during a given cycle. It wasn't until I talked to my colleagues who also study women's cycles that I realized this was normal. Most researchers who study ovulation fail to find evidence of ovulation in about 30 to 35 percent of their sample. This is true despite the fact that our samples are comprised exclusively of young, healthy women with no endocrinological disorders and regular periods.

The reason women experience so much variation in hormone production across cycles is because pregnancy isn't always a good idea. And our bodies know that. And because of that, the functioning of our brain-ovarian axis (the communication pathway between the brain and our ovaries) is exquisitely sensitive to stress. The stress can come from pressures at work, school, or home; lack of social support; not getting enough calories or having nutritional deficiencies; illness, inflammation, or vaccines* . . . it can come from anywhere. Anything that engages the body's stress response for prolonged periods of time (including even seasonal stress caused by wintertime!) can send signals to the brain that pregnancy is a bad idea. And when our brain receives enough of these signals, it will shut down ovulation until things improve. This is true for humans. This is true for our nonhuman primate relatives. This is true for other nonprimate mammals. Stressed-out mammalian females do not like to ovulate. And nonovulatory cycles create hormone imbalances characterized by high levels of estrogen and low or absent levels of progesterone.

---

* This does *not* mean that vaccines are bad! They're not! Research finds that any disruption or delay in ovulation from vaccines is short-lived and will resolve as soon at the immunological response to the vaccine is over. You might not want to plan on trying to conceive or retrieve eggs for IVF or egg freezing during a cycle when getting a vaccination, but getting vaccines has no lasting effect on fertility (and, if anything, might have a positive effect in the long term since it will decrease your probability of ovulation suppression from acute illness or disease).

Thankfully, there are a number of things that you can do to support your cycle and help promote balance between estrogen and progesterone. Happily, these activities also have the effect of increasing your resilience to hormonal changes across the cycle and can put an end to PMS. Hormonal balance and resilience are all about creating a body that feels safe, healthy, and well nourished enough to ovulate. They're also about promoting the sort of cellular plasticity that helps minimize the physiological turbulence caused by hormonal change.

We're going to spend the rest of this chapter talking about what you can do to achieve these things. And as you'll see, it's a lot easier than you might think.

Supporting Ovulation and Resilience to Hormonal Changes

I'm going to start with the good news. You don't need to do anything overly complicated or expensive to support ovulation and resilience to hormonal changes. You don't need to buy overpriced supplements, you don't need special equipment, you don't need a ten-day juice cleanse . . . There is no need to turn your life totally upside down or bankrupt yourself to support your cycle and eliminate PMS. The things that will have the biggest impact on your cycle—both your hormone production and having a luteal phase that doesn't make you feel like sh*t—are so accessible to all of us that they're practically boring. Whether you regularly ovulate and how quickly your cells can adapt to hormonal change has nothing to do with how many potions you're willing to choke down or the timing of your last cleanse. Instead, they have everything to do with what you're eating, whether you exercise, and the steps you take to manage stress, get sleep, stay connected, and limit your exposure to toxins.

That's the good news.

The bad news is that these things are far easier said than done. It can be hard for us to know where to start when it comes to eating well and getting ourselves on track with sleep and exercise when we have a lot of changes to make. It can also feel confusing when there is so much conflicting information out there. It can be tempting to want to buy magical potions and elixirs that promise quick solutions to hormonal balance because it allows us to tune out the noise and avoid the guesswork of figuring all of this out on our own.

Thankfully, when you look at what science has to say about supporting hormonal balance and resilience, you'll see that it's a relatively uncomplicated set of recommendations. The pillars of hormonal health are more or less unchanged from what they were for our distant female ancestors. To ovulate regularly and be resilient to the physiological chaos resulting from hormonal change, our bodies need to:

- be well nourished
- be well rested
- be active
- manage stress well
- have meaningful connections with other people, and
- avoid chemicals that f*ck up our hormones.

In the sections that follow, we will go over what research tells us about the role of nutrition, exercise, and other lifestyle factors in promoting hormonal balance and resilience. Then I will offer you practical solutions to make these lifestyle changes accessible and doable—health hacks I've developed and fine-tuned so I can support my health while also being present for my family and building my career. I have had to learn through trial and error what works and what doesn't while not making my health its own full-time job.

Nutrition

Let's start by talking about nutrition. We're starting here because what you eat is hands down one of the most important influencers of health (if not *the* most important influencer). A ton of research shows that when your body is in good health, it promotes regular ovulation and fewer PMS symptoms. Women who regularly eat processed foods have a prevalence of PMS that is almost three times higher than those who regularly consume whole, unprocessed foods. That's an almost 200 percent increased risk! Other research finds that women's healthy eating scores (a score calculated by comparing the relative ratios of whole, unprocessed foods to fast and processed foods) predict lower depression and anxiety in the luteal phase as well as better sleep. If there is only one recommendation that I could make to enhance women's experiences in the luteal phase, it would be to improve the quality of your diet. It makes such a huge difference in how women experience their hormonal changes across the cycle.

So, what does healthy eating look like? Well, the preponderance of the evidence in nutrition science suggests that . . . drum roll, please . . . there is no research consensus on what the healthiest diet is for the human body. Systematic reviews of the literature examining the health impacts of multiple types of diets done by the best and the brightest in the world of nutrition science conclude that there is no one healthy eating practice that is best. But what's clear is that any diet that (a) is made up of whole-food sources (meaning unprocessed foods that your great-great-great-grandmother would recognize) and (b) emphasizes plants is going to help optimize health. And this is true whether it takes the form of a Mediterranean diet, a plant-based diet, a ketogenic diet, a Paleo diet . . . or whatever mode of eating it is that you prefer.

When you consider the range of foods that our ancestors survived on, this actually makes a lot of sense. Our bodies are made to thrive on whole foods that exist in nature, but beyond that, it would have been disadvantageous to be too picky. Can you imagine one of our distant ancestors walking miles across the African savanna in search of food and then, at the end of the day, being offered a meal made of starchy tubers and saying, "No thank you, I am keto"? Our bodies are optimized for eating a range of whole foods, but the specifics of what foods matter far less than having a general emphasis on:

- Limiting or avoiding refined starches like flour
- Limiting or avoiding added sugars

- Limiting or avoiding processed foods (most of which contain flour and added sugar, along with a whole bunch of other nonsense your body doesn't need)
- Emphasizing whole, plant-based foods
- If animal protein is included, focusing on lean red meats, fish, eggs, poultry, and seafood raised eating native diets and (ideally) living in conditions similar to their natural habitats

If you eat a diet that follows these general guiding principles—which are best summarized by Michael Pollan in his wonderful essays and books on food as "Eat food, not too much, mostly plants"—you will be doing all that is required of you to support hormonal health. There is no special set of rules that you need to follow to have healthy hormones and promote resilience to hormonal changes.

I feel best eating a mostly plant-based diet with well-sourced animal protein* thrown in maybe once or twice a week. My blood work is best, and I feel best when I eat this way. Some weeks, I eat no animal products at all; some weeks, I will have multiple servings. I honestly don't think about it too much because I like to keep things simple. I just use the principles listed above to guide my food choices. As a result, my meals are generally made up of foods that my great-great-grandmother would recognize (minus dairy†). This is how I feel best, perform best, and it is what supports my blood work being in optimal range.

You may be different. You may feel best eating exclusively plant-based, keto, Paleo, or Mediterranean. The good news about adopting a simple set of healthy eating guidelines is that it allows you to experiment and to eat to your tastes, your budget, and according to the seasons and food availability. I encourage you to monitor your

---

* Things like cage-free eggs, wild-caught fish, or the meat from animals eating their traditional diets (like grass-raised beef or wild-caught venison).

† But even with this, I am not super strict. If I want to take my kids out for ice cream, we go out for ice cream . . . and I eat it and enjoy it. Because this is something that we do maybe three or four times a year, it's not something I spend too much time thinking about. Individual behaviors matter so much less than habits.

own reactions to foods to see which form of healthful eating allows your body to feel its best and proceed from there. Regardless of what anyone might try to tell you, there is no—and I repeat *no*—consensus on what the best diet is, so there is room for experimentation. As long as you stick to the rules outlined above, you can make personalized adjustments that make your body feel best.

Even though there are a lot of people who make money from confusion over nutrition, the fact is, healthy eating really isn't complicated. It's just hard to do. Most of the edible products that masquerade as food in the developed world do not nourish our bodies and are engineered to be addictive and create cravings. And because of this, research finds that the biggest barrier to healthy eating isn't lack of information about what's healthy and what's not (junk food is like pornography: you know it when you see it), it's about knowing how to translate those principles into sustainable practices that keep us well fed and well nourished in the face of a food landscape filled with addictive foods and a lot of fad diet noise.

Here are a few simple habits that I have found to be tremendously helpful in setting up my life in a way that promotes healthy eating. Although I am far from perfect, anyone who knows me will tell you that I practice what I preach when it comes to good nutrition most of the time. I'm sharing what I learned in the hopes that it may help you with your own healthy eating goals.

- Embrace preparing food. Although there are food preparation services you can use to create health-promoting meals and snacks with minimal effort, these can be expensive and out of most people's reach. Because of this, if you are going to eat foods that fuel your body and support hormonal health, you are going to need to embrace the art of food preparation. This is something that you have time to do, even if you think you're too busy.* You just need to lean

---

* Except in rare circumstances, this is true. My schedule is insane but I still find time to prepare food because I make it a priority.

into the fact that chopping things up in the kitchen is going to be part of the way you spend your time from now on. I know it's a pain, but I promise you that it is worth it. The time you spend in the kitchen is going to pay you back with improved health, better energy, less turbulence across the cycle, and hormonal balance. And, as an added bonus, it counts as physical activity. I get in an extra three to four thousand or so steps* on days that I spend time cooking dinner and packing lunches at night. I have come to really enjoy the time I spend preparing food, especially when I think about it as also being an opportunity to keep my body active. Even if you don't love it at first, coming to terms with the fact that you are going to have to spend time preparing food is the first step toward shifting your life toward one that embraces good nutrition.

- Find some cookbooks or cooking websites that take a health- or nourishment-forward approach to food and pick some recipes to start with. I have included some of my favorite recipe books and websites in appendix D in case you need help getting started. Start by bookmarking recipes that look tasty to you and then pick one or two that you will cook this week. If you are new to cooking, start with something that looks good and doesn't require too many ingredients. It's easy to get overwhelmed and decide cooking sucks if you choose a recipe with a giant list of ingredients that requires you to spend two or more hours measuring and chopping before you even pull out a pan. Another note for new cooks: Know that you need to prep all the ingredients for your dish *before* you start cooking

---

* If you clock in less than this, here is my hot tip to increase your step count: be hopelessly disorganized. As a fairly disorganized home cook, I am constantly having to run back and forth to the pantry, refrigerator, spice drawer, etc., to fetch things as I go. You too can increase your physical activity one forgotten saucepan at a time. You're welcome.

anything. When I first started cooking, I was miserable and nothing turned out right because I was prepping as I cooked. Buy a handful of small ramekin dishes from your favorite kitchen store or Amazon so that you have a place to put the ingredients that you chop and measure to have ready to go before you actually start cooking.

- Once you have a recipe you like, make extra in the future for leftovers or lunches the next day. This makes meal planning much easier and minimizes time spent cooking while maximizing time spent eating home-cooked food.
- If you work outside the home full time like I do, consider using your weekend to plan your dinner menus for the week and purchase all or most of the groceries so you are well stocked for the week and have everything on hand that you need. Make sure your grocery list includes all the ingredients for the meals you'll cook for dinner as well as whatever you need for breakfast and lunch.
- Pick a day each week to (a) chop up veggies that you can eat as snacks for the week (peppers, carrots, radishes, sugar snap peas, cucumbers, mushrooms, cauliflower, and fennel bulb are my go-to snacky veggies) and (b) do as much advance meal prep for the week as you are able to stomach. If your work schedule looks like mine, this will probably be something you want to do on a Saturday or Sunday. Even though it can feel less than thrilling to be chopping vegetables and prepping food over the weekend, Future You will be so thankful for the effort when she goes to the refrigerator to prepare dinner or throw together a quick lunch and finds that everything is ready. Future Sarah is always so thankful for the efforts of Past Sarah when she grabs her prepped veggies from the fridge during the week. You can do as much or as little advance work as you want. When my kids were little, I would spend the whole first half of the day on Sundays chopping, measuring, prepping, and putting things into glass storage containers to use through-

out the week. I still do a fair amount of that now (if you come to my house, you will see that all my veggies are chopped and in storage containers by the end of day Sunday), but I no longer have to measure out the ingredients I need for recipes I plan to cook during the week ahead of time. Now that my kids are older and don't want my constant attention before we sit down to eat, I have more time to cook at a leisurely pace when I get home from work.

- Don't feel like you need to do everything perfectly and allow yourself to ease into it. If you are not used to preparing your own food, start small. Plan on cooking one or two dinners using whole-food ingredients during the week. You can gradually increase the number of meals you prepare from scratch as you get more endurance. (I know that seems like an odd word to use to describe what's required with food preparation, but that really is what it takes.) I know it can feel like a beatdown to cook after a very long day at work, but it can become really enjoyable if you use it as a time to unwind and listen to a podcast, the evening news, or your favorite music. I look forward to coming home, putting on my yoga pants, and preparing food that I love. I look at it as an opportunity to be physically active, do something health promoting for myself and my family, and listen to whatever music I want without apology. It is the time when I transition between the office and home life and I really value having that hour to myself with just me, my favorite music, and foods I love.
- Have one or two go-to things that you have for breakfast and lunch most days so that you're not constantly having to think about what you're going to eat. Ideally, these will be made with whole foods, are filling, and are easy to make. This will make everything so much easier with your grocery shopping and help you stay on track with eating well. You may want to experiment with some different breakfast and lunch recipes before landing on something

that you can eat most days without getting bored. Then, plan on eating those things most days. For me, there are about three things I eat for breakfast, and my lunch is either leftovers from dinner the night before or a big salad that's loaded with veggies, tofu, different types of beans, nuts, seeds, avocado, and red or white wine vinegar.

- Keep addictive "food" out of the house to the extent that it is possible. I have food in quotes because hyperpalatable foodstuff (that ultraprocessed nonsense that pretends to be food) hardly fits the definition of what food is supposed to be. It isn't nourishing. It isn't filling. And it's made to be addictive. It shouldn't qualify as food. This doesn't mean that you can't have anything in your house that is there just for pleasure (at any moment, you will find my house stocked with dark chocolate and homemade baked goods). You just don't want to be surrounded by addictive foods, because they are, well, addictive, not nourishing, and are not promoting your health. Eating for pleasure is a wonderful thing. Eating because the thing you are consuming has been engineered to make you want to eat more is not.

Eating foods that nourish your body will help decrease inflammation, increase cellular plasticity, and help keep your body at a healthy weight. Each of these outcomes is associated with more resilience to hormonal changes and fewer PMS symptoms. It will also help support healthy ovulation, making it a win-win.

> **WHAT IS SEED CYCLING AND DO I NEED TO DO IT?**
>
> When you get into the health and wellness space and start talking about nutrition for healthy cycles, you will often hear about the practice of seed cycling. This is when you eat specific types of seeds during different phases of the menstrual cycle to help balance hormone levels and support reproductive

health. The idea is that certain seeds contain nutrients and compounds that can promote estrogen or progesterone production at the appropriate time in the cycle. Although there is limited scientific evidence to support its effectiveness (and it's not something I do), I know women who swear that it helps smooth out their cycles. So, in case you're interested in trying it, here's how it works:

Follicular Phase (Days 1–14-ish):

- **Seeds used:** Flaxseeds and pumpkin seeds
- **Purpose:** Support and balance estrogen

  Flaxseeds contain lignans, which are phytoestrogens that can help modulate estrogen levels, either supporting the body's natural estrogen production or binding excess estrogen to prevent hormonal imbalance.

  Pumpkin seeds are rich in zinc, which is believed to support the release of progesterone during the luteal phase.

- **How to use:** Typically, 1–2 tablespoons of each seed are consumed daily, ground to improve nutrient absorption.

Luteal Phase (Days 15–28-ish):

- **Seeds used:** Sesame seeds and sunflower seeds
- **Purpose:** Support progesterone and balance estrogen

  Sesame seeds also contain lignans that help balance estrogen levels, and they are rich in magnesium and zinc, which are thought to support progesterone production.

Sunflower seeds are high in vitamin E and selenium, both of which are believed to support luteal-phase hormone production and promote progesterone levels.

- **How to use:** Again, 1–2 tablespoons of each seed are consumed daily, ground for better absorption.

How Seed Cycling Is Supposed to Support the Menstrual Cycle

- **Hormonal balance:** The different seeds used in each phase are rich in nutrients that are thought to support the production of key hormones. Flaxseeds and sesame seeds are particularly noted for containing lignans, which can help balance estrogen. Sunflower seeds and pumpkin seeds contain zinc, magnesium, selenium, and vitamin E, which are believed to support progesterone production.

- **Support for estrogen detoxification:** The fiber in flaxseeds and sesame seeds is thought to help with the detoxification of excess estrogen by helping you poop, which is important for hormonal balance.

Does it work? It's hard to tell. Like I said, there really isn't much research evidence either supporting or refuting this practice. If you are interested in trying it, why not? It certainly can't hurt. I love putting these seeds in my oatmeal and on my salads on all days of the month because I think they're really tasty, add interesting texture, and have a ton of great micronutrients. If nothing else, you'll give yourself a vitamin boost and some new flavors to experiment with.

Movement

The second thing you can do to promote healthy cycles and resilience to hormonal changes is . . . drum roll, please . . . exercise. Because as boring as it is to hear, research finds that exercise can really, *really* make a difference in how you feel as your hormones shift across the cycle. The positive impact that physical activity has on mood—both in the luteal phase and outside of it—is inarguable. Exercise is regularly found to be *at least as effective* as antidepressants at improving mood, and its side effects are far more tolerable. Antidepressant side effects include things like genital numbness and lack of sexual desire. Exercise side effects include things like looking smokin' hotttt and preventing chronic disease . . . I mean, is there even a contest???

The reason exercise is such a powerful feel-good drug is because it flips switches from head to toe that help stabilize mood and promote well-being. It decreases mood-ruining inflammation. It increases the functioning of neurotransmitter systems in the brain that regulate and stabilize mood. It increases neuroplasticity (which slows cognitive decline, keeps our brain sharp, and stabilizes mood by allowing our cells to gracefully adjust to changing levels of sex hormones). It also increases blood flow to the brain, which keeps the cells happy and adaptable to change and keeps us feeling confident, alert, and ready to cope with challenges.

Not surprisingly, regular physical activity is found to predict less PMS and more regular ovulation than what is observed in nonexercisers. Although really high-intensity exercise can mess with ovulation if you don't compensate with increased food intake, the level of exercise that most of us do is helpful, not harmful, to regular ovulation. So if you are hoping to take the edge off PMS and support healthy hormone production, consider adding more physical activity to your life. This can look like whatever you want it to. You just need to move. I do resistance training and intense cardio in the follicular phase, yoga in the luteal phase, and other things to keep myself active (horseback riding, riding my bike, cooking dinner, and daily walks) throughout.

If you don't know where to start, just lace up your sneakers and go outside for a walk. If it's cold, bundle up. If it's hot, go early in the morning before the sun comes up. Every step you take (literally) to improve the amount of activity your body does every day will help get you on the path to a better luteal phase.

Sleep

Another way we can support our hormonal health and balance is by getting more sleep. Research finds that getting good sleep decreases negative premenstrual symptoms and helps promote fertility and hormone production. It does this by improving cognitive control over our emotions (which is when we are able to talk ourselves out of feeling bad about something), raising the threshold for emotional activation (meaning that we're able to put up with more nonsense before losing our cool), increasing neuroplasticity (keeping our brain nimble and able to roll with the punches), and supporting regular ovulation. Trying to aim for a solid seven-plus hours of sleep each night is a good place to start to help support ovulation and resilience to hormonal changes. Although women are more likely to experience sleep disturbances in the luteal phase of the cycle than the follicular (this is hypothesized to be related to decreased melatonin secretion in response to luteal-phase hormonal changes), you can help improve your sleep in and out of the luteal phase by:

- Reducing caffeine and alcohol (especially later in the day when they are more likely to disrupt sleep).
- Staying physically active (physical exhaustion is an amazing sleep aid).
- Getting outdoor light in the morning to help set your circadian clocks. Regular exposure to direct sunlight—particularly in the morning—helps synchronize the body's internal clock with the external day-night cycle, supporting better sleep and overall health. Getting sunlight on your

skin also helps the body synthesize vitamin D, which supports ovulation and can reduce PMS.
- Wearing blue-light-blocking glasses when looking at screens in the late afternoon and evening hours. Yes, these glasses can look ridiculous, but they are great for promoting healthy circadian rhythms and sleep. Blue light—which is present in sunlight but also in the artificial light emitted from phone, computer, and television screens—enters the retina and goes into the suprachiasmatic nucleus (the SCN, which is the master circadian clock in the brain), telling your brain it's daytime. This can suppress melatonin production and make it more difficult for us to fall asleep. It is also worth noting that artificial light at inappropriate times (for example, looking at computer screens at night) can negatively impact ovulation and reproductive function. For example, in one cohort study that included more than seventy-one thousand reproductive-age women, researchers found that night-shift work was associated with an increased probability of having cycle irregularities, which are often a product of ovulatory disturbances. And one other recent systematic review that included a meta-analysis of sixty-two studies found that night-shift work is associated with a 23 percent increased risk of miscarriage, a 13 percent increase in the rate of preterm birth, and an 18 percent increase risk of having a small-for-gestational-age newborn, demonstrating that these effects on reproductive function can persist throughout gestation.
- Establishing a predictable sleep routine. For me, this means making a lavender or valerian tea and reading, sometimes after a hot bath. Getting into a healthy sleep routine helps cue your brain that it's time to start closing up shop and get ready to shift gears into sleep mode.

Quit Smoking and Reconsider Alcohol

Drinking less or avoiding alcohol altogether and quitting smoking can also improve your resilience to hormonal changes and promote healthy ovulation. Although you undoubtedly know that smoking is linked to health problems like lung cancer and emphysema, you might not know that it also elevates inflammation (which increases your risk of pretty much everything that can go wrong in the human body), worsens PMS, and can disrupt ovulation. So if you are a smoker, please quit. It's terrible for your health, and there are so many resources available that can help ease you out of the habit. It is far less painful to quit smoking than it used to be and your luteal-phase hormones can help. Progesterone decreases the reward value of substances like nicotine, alcohol, and other drugs, making the luteal phase a great time to walk away from substances that no longer serve you.

Alcohol isn't great for hormonal health either. Research finds that drinking alcohol may be linked to a worse premenstrual mood and disrupted ovulation. In one recent study, researchers pooled data from nineteen different studies that included more than forty-seven thousand participants across eight different countries. When looking at the relationship between alcohol consumption and PMS, they found that drinking moderate amounts of alcohol (here defined as consumption of one drink per day) increased women's risk of PMS by 45 percent. And heavy drinkers—those who averaged greater than one drink per day—increased their risk of PMS by 79 percent. Although these studies aren't able to establish a cause-and-effect relationship between alcohol intake and PMS, the consistency of these results suggests that alcohol intake is probably not great for PMS. Limiting or abstaining from alcohol is health promoting and improves the quality of sleep, making the decision to skip drinks before dinner one that will likely improve your mood symptoms in the luteal phase.

Another reason to consider decreasing or abstaining from alcohol is that it may interfere with ovulation and healthy hormone production. Although there hasn't been a great deal of research on alcohol intake and failure to ovulate or hormone production per se, there has been quite a bit of evidence suggesting that alcohol intake can interfere with conception, suggesting that alcohol may negatively impact ovulation and hormone production. For example, in one study, researchers found that heavy alcohol use (here defined as more than six drinks per week) at any point in the cycle was associated with reduced odds of conception relative to women who did not consume alcohol. They also found that even moderate alcohol intake (here defined as three to six drinks per week), when it occurred in the luteal phase, predicted a lowered likelihood of conception compared to what was observed in nondrinkers, suggesting that our cycles may be more sensitive to the effects of alcohol in the luteal phase than in the follicular. These results were echoed in a recent research review examining studies measuring the links between alcohol intake and fecundability (biologyspeak for the probability of getting pregnant within the course of a single cycle). They found that light drinkers' fecundability was 89 percent of that of their nondrinking peers, and that moderate to heavy drinkers' fecundability was only 77 percent of that of their nondrinking peers.

Although you will be hard-pressed to find research that demonstrates an inarguable cause-and-effect relationship between alcohol intake and PMS or alcohol intake and lowered fecundability, there is no research that finds the opposite relationship. There are no studies published (at least none that I have seen) that find that mood and/or fecundability are higher in alcohol drinkers compared to nondrinkers. This alone should let you know that alcohol is probably no friend to your hormones and ability to navigate hormonal change.

When we consider all the things that alcohol does to the body, this makes perfect sense. It disrupts sleep, lowers heart-rate variability (which decreases your body's resilience to stress), and decreases your liver's ability to metabolize sex hormones because it's tied up metabolizing that predinner martini. None of these things are doing your mood any favors in the luteal phase or helping out egg development, making alcohol something that should be minimized or abstained from if you are trying to improve your luteal-phase mood and promote healthy hormone release.

Managing Stress

Most women I know vastly underestimate the importance of stress management in their body's resilience to hormonal changes and sex-hormone production. And at the risk of sounding like the president of the tinfoil hat society, I think this is information intentionally kept from us. There are a lot of people who have a vested interest in keeping women stressed to the max and neglecting ourselves in the name of free labor. Our employers, our kids' schools, our kids' extracurricular activities, and every other organization that runs off of women's unpaid contributions of time and effort win when we ignore our need to unwind and take time for self-care. There are a lot of jobs that wouldn't get done and businesses that would cease to exist if women collectively chose to walk away from all of the unnecessary demands on their time and decided to invest in taking care of themselves instead. There are a lot of people who benefit from the fact that we've all somehow come to the agreement that the only way to be a good employee or parent or group member is to completely neglect our own needs for the needs of others and treat our need for downtime as a character flaw.

And this should really p*ss you off.

Even though there isn't much noise made about the importance of stress management to our health and hormone production, it is incredibly important to both. Managing our stress and having meaningful relationships with others helps keep inflammation low, supercharges the immune system, promotes healthy functioning of the HPA axis (your brain-stress axis), and promotes the release of feel-good neurotransmitters. All these things improve our body's ability to roll with the punches when our hormones change rapidly like they do in the luteal phase. And because of this, having healthy relationships, social support, and being on top of our stress management game are all linked to having less psychological turbulence in the luteal phase and less PMS.

Stress management is also incredibly important for ovulation and hormone production. As we have talked about many times now in the book, your body will turn ovulation off like a light switch if it suspects that pregnancy is a bad idea. And stress is generally a good indicator that things aren't going great, which is why research regularly finds that chronic stress is linked with failure to ovulate, infertility, and hormone dysregulation. In one recent study, researchers found that women who reported higher levels of daily stress had higher rates of failed ovulation and lower hormone levels than women who reported lower levels of daily stress. Specifically, they found that for each unit increase in these women's levels of daily stress, they had 70 percent higher odds of failing to ovulate. *Seventy percent higher odds!!* They also found these women's levels of sex hormones to be lower, which is what you'd expect when ovulation is compromised.

Our cycles are incredibly sensitive to stress and other cues that provide the brain with information about the wisdom of pregnancy. And because stress and social isolation are potent cues of conditions not being optimal for pregnancy, these are often potent ovulation suppressors as well. For example, researchers in one study of 154 women who were in an intense three-year nursing program at a military institution in South Korea found that an overwhelming majority of them (69.9 percent!!) had nonovulatory cycles during the school months. Similar patterns were observed around the globe during the SARS-CoV-2 (COVID-19) pandemic, with researchers finding that 63 percent of their sample experienced suppressed ovulation at this time. In this latter study, the researchers also found that the women who had ovulatory disturbances were those who experienced greater feelings of frustration, anxiety, isolation, depression, and outside stress during this period than did the 37 percent of women whose ovulation was not disturbed.

Mechanistically, this works because of the antagonistic relationship between stress hormones and sex hormones. When stress hormones like cortisol are high, it blocks the secretion and action of the gonadotropin-releasing hormones (GnRH) whose job it is (via the pituitary gland) to tell the ovaries to mature egg follicles and ovulate. Essentially, when the brain is stressed, it won't tell the ovaries to ovulate, inhibiting egg development and ovulation until conditions improve. There is also some research that finds stress in the follicular phase can disrupt ovulation through the adrenal release of progesterone (which is something male and female bodies both do in response to stress), suggesting that stress occurring at any point in the cycle can delay or disrupt ovulation. Finding a way to manage your stress is important for promoting ovulation and healthy hormone production because too much stress disrupts ovulation.

When you look at research on the incidence of overwhelming stress in women, it's clear that we have a lot of work to do in this area. We are facing an epidemic of chronic stress. Research finds that nearly 69 percent of women in the United States report stress levels above what is considered healthy. Stress management is something we all need to take more seriously than most of us do because too much stress is all that most of us have ever known. We have to unlearn the belief that our value is tied up in our productivity and that we've failed if we aren't competitive in six different sports and can't speak conversational Mandarin because (a) this simply isn't true, and (b) these beliefs are bad for our health, hormone production, and fertility.

The good news is, taking steps to improve your stress and social connectedness to others will usually completely reverse ovulation suppression. In one recent study, researchers tested whether cognitive behavioral therapy (CBT) would help women with functional hypothalamic amenorrhea (where the body shuts down ovarian function in response to some sort of stress) get their cycles back. To test this, they had women participate in sixteen sessions of cognitive behavioral therapy that took place over twenty weeks. The sessions focused on stress-management techniques and adopting healthy attitudes about exercise, nutrition, and weight. The women exposed to CBT (compared to the control group, which did not get therapy) experienced a decrease in cortisol levels and, for many of them, ovulation resumed.

In addition to CBT, here are other measures that research finds to be effective in helping lower stress and (in turn) promoting resilience to hormonal changes and healthy ovulation:

- **Mindfulness-based stress reduction (MBSR).** This is a type of mindfulness practice that aims to enhance the ability to observe (rather than react to) stressful events. It works by training the mind to focus on the immediate content of stressful experiences and to recognize that our reactions to these events are temporary and not diagnostic of some larger truth (the whole feelings-are-not-facts paradigm). Although this sort of practice can be done in a variety of different ways, they all focus on changing our tendency to experience knee-jerk emotional reactions to stress and then ruminate about them. And it seems to work. Research finds MBSR interventions to be effective at reducing stress, depression, and anxiety symptoms. Although I haven't seen any studies looking at the effectiveness of MBSR at promoting healthy ovulation or minimizing symptoms of PMS, given its proven ability to reduce stress and improve mental health, I would be hugely surprised if it wasn't therapeutic in this context as well.
- **Exercise.** I am sure that you are tired of hearing about it by now, but research finds that regular physical activity is consistently shown to lower stress, reduce symptoms of anxiety and depression, and improve resilience to future stressors. It also improves mood, cognitive function, and sleep, all of which can lower stress.
- **Social support.** Engaging with friends, family, or support groups can provide emotional support and help individuals cope with stress. Positive social connections act as a buffer against stress.
- **Expressive writing.** Writing about stressful experiences helps people process their emotions and reflect on ways to

manage stress more effectively. Studies show that expressive writing reduces stress, enhances mental well-being, and can even improve immune function.

Limit Exposure to Endocrine Disrupters

Limit exposure to endocrine-disrupting compounds (EDCs), which are chemicals that can mimic, block, or alter the normal functioning of hormones. You can find EDCs in lots of different types of products, including pesticides, plastics, personal-care products, and industrial chemicals. Although there isn't a ton of research on the effects of EDCs on PMS or ovulatory function in humans, they're called endocrine disrupters for a reason. It's a good idea to try to minimize your exposure if you're hoping to have a happy, healthy cycle. If you are looking for somewhere to start, here is a list of some products that frequently contain EDCs, along with some notes about what to do to help minimize exposures:

- Plastic containers (Look for those saying BPA-free or free of phthalates.)
- Personal-care products (Look for shampoos, lotions, and cosmetics that are free of parabens and phthalates.)
- Pesticides (Look for all-natural products that are free of DDT or atrazine.)
- Canned foods (Most contain BPA and other endocrine disrupters in their lining; opt for frozen or shelf-stable foods stored in boxes.)
- Household cleaning products (Look for products that do not contain chemicals like alkylphenols.)
- Nonstick cookware (These often contain PFOA or PFAS, both of which are endocrine disrupting, so use stainless-steel pots or cast-iron pans instead.)
- Flame retardants (These are found in furniture and elec-

tronics with PBDEs; ask your retailer what is in the products you would like to buy.)
- Detergents (Look for natural products that do not contain nonylphenol ethoxylates.)
- Fragranced products (Anything containing synthetic musks can be endocrine disrupting, although natural oils can mess up hormones too. It is better to be scent free for hormone health.)

Now, before you freak out and start throwing away everything you own that contains either plastic or a scent, I want to point out that limiting exposure to EDCs helps promote hormonal health, but this shouldn't be the primary focus of your efforts if you are looking to improve hormonal balance and resilience. It matters, but it matters less than some of the other things we have talked about. Sometimes I'll see people frantically obsess over what's in their face cream or freaking out about the fact that they can't afford a sustainably sourced, organic couch, but the same people don't spend any time getting sunlight, exercising, or nourishing their bodies with health-supporting foods. If this describes you, know that I am saying this with all the compassion and kindness in the world, but research suggests that your energy may be misplaced. Nourishing, moving, and resting our bodies are the pillars of hormonal resilience, regular cycles, and health. Doing these things is more important than what is—or is not—in your face cream. So while I definitely recommend avoiding endocrine disrupters to the extent that you are able to do so, it's probably not necessary to get rid of all your worldly possessions or start making your own shampoo to have healthy hormones.

When our bodies are well nourished and don't have excess body fat, they're actually decently efficient at clearing EDCs and minimizing their impact on our health. This does *not* mean that these compounds are okay for us and we shouldn't try to avoid them when possible. Instead, it means that the effects of these compounds on our bodies are much less pronounced when we are well nourished and do not have excess body fat than they are when we do. Eating a plant-rich diet increases intake of natural detoxifying agents such as allicin, quercetin, sulforaphane, and anthocyanin (found in fruits and vegetables like blueberries, onions, broccoli, brussels sprouts, and cauliflower), which help your body clear EDCs before they can wreak havoc on your hormones. And keeping excess body fat at bay will prevent these compounds (most of which are fat soluble) from sticking around in your body longer than they should. Making time in your schedule to be sure that you are maintaining the pillars of good health (nourishment and movement, in particular) will help minimize the impact of EDCs on your body if you have an accidental perfume relapse or don't have control over your exposures.

How Do I Know If I'm Ovulating?

One of the most important things you can do to help monitor your hormonal health is to keep tabs on whether you are ovulating. Most people assume that if they have regular periods they are ovulating regularly, but as we've seen, this isn't necessarily true. Many studies that track women's ovulation find failure to ovulate both common and difficult to notice. Many times, women's nonovulatory cycles are virtually indistinguishable from those in which ovulation actually occurred. You can't just assume that if you got your period and your cycle was the same length as it always is that you've ovulated. You have to learn how to read your body's cues to get a better picture of what's happening.

How do you tell whether you've ovulated? The first thing that you need to do is start tracking your cycle (I know . . . it's my answer for everything, but honestly it's the only way to know). Each day, make note of (a) your basal body temperature (which you can track using wearable tech or measure yourself using a digital thermometer first thing after waking up), (b) your cervical mucus, and (c) your cervical position. In the box on pages 206–7, I give you instructions on how to keep tabs on what's going on with your cervix in case you've never interacted with it before. And in the back of the book (see appendix A), I have links to free cycle-tracking resources if you don't want to have to make your own cycle-tracking chart from scratch. This should be pretty much everything you need to start keeping track of your fertility today.

Here's what you can expect to find:

In the early follicular phase (when you have your period and soon after it's done), your cervix should be low, firm, and mostly or completely closed. You will also have a relatively low amount of cervical mucus at this time and your body temperature will be relatively low (your temperature will drop between 0.5 and 1 degree Fahrenheit just prior to getting your period . . . this is always my cue to grab a handful of tampons to stick in my purse).

The next thing that will happen is that the mucus around your cervix will become increasingly abundant and wet as you begin to approach the fertile window. This is something that happens to make the area more hospitable to sperm and gives you a sign that your estrogen levels are increasing. As you approach ovulation (usually around Day 14), your cervix should feel soft (kind of like touching your lips), it will be higher up (it can be harder to find near ovulation), and the mucus should be slippery, clear, and increasingly abundant.[*] This is the first clue that you are going to ovulate or are in the process of ovulating.

---

[*] Some women also experience a slight dip in temperature accompanying ovulation, but it often isn't detectable with a thermometer or health tech (Oura Ring, Apple Watch, etc.), and it's highly variable both within and between women.

STEPS TO FEEL YOUR CERVIX AND EXAMINE CERVICAL MUCUS

1. Wash your hands so that you don't introduce any unwanted bacteria into your vaginal canal.

2. Find a comfortable position: You can either squat, sit on the toilet, or put one leg up on a surface like the edge of your bathtub, the toilet seat, or the park bench at your favorite public space (kidding!).

3. Insert your middle finger into your vagina and gently reach upward. You should feel your cervix at the end of the vaginal canal. It will feel sort of like a small, firm, rounded nub.

4. Note the position and texture:
   - During ovulation, the cervix tends to be soft, high, open, and wet (kind of like what it feels like when you touch your lips).
   - Outside of ovulation, the cervix is usually firmer, lower, closed, and dry (kind of what it feels like to touch the tip of your nose).

Things You Might Feel Near Ovulation

- High cervix: During ovulation, the cervix is positioned higher, making it harder to reach.
- Softness: It becomes softer during fertile days.
- Opening: The cervix opens slightly to allow sperm to pass through when ovulating.

Cervical mucus is easy to track once you've already had your finger(s) all up in your business. Simply examine what you pull out:

- If it is wet, clear and slippery like egg whites, and abundant, this is fertile mucus and will be present in the days leading up to ovulation (and on the day of ovulation itself).

- If it is thick, sticky, and white, this generally means that ovulation has already occurred, and you are in the luteal phase.

Remember to track these changes over time to become more familiar with how your cervix feels at different points in your cycle.

When you are anticipating ovulation, you can also use a luteinizing hormone (LH) test if you want to verify that ovulation is forthcoming. Luteinizing hormone surges twelve to thirty-six hours before ovulation and triggers the release of an egg from the ovary. If you measure LH (which you can do with a simple at-home urine test) and get a positive result, it generally means that you're going to ovulate in the next day or so.

If you want to use an at-home LH test to tell whether you are going to ovulate, start testing a few days before you expect ovulation to happen. If you have a twenty-eight-day cycle, I would start testing around Day 10 or 11 and continue testing until you detect the surge. Although LH tests are often heralded as the gold standard for estimating ovulation, they have a pretty high rate of false negatives. This means that it isn't unusual for women to get a negative LH test, but then ovulate anyway. For this reason, I would only recommend LH testing when used in conjunction with other tracking metrics like your temperature and cervical position and mucus. Relying on LH tests as a way to track ovulation—in addition to getting expensive after a while—isn't necessarily going to give you an accurate read on your fertility.

After the fertile window has passed, the next thing you want to look for is evidence that ovulation has occurred. The first clue most women generally get is a rise in body temperature. As we've talked about a few times, your body temperature increases almost a full degree (Fahrenheit) when progesterone begins to rise. Generally, women experience a shift in body temperature twelve to twenty-four hours after ovulation has occurred. Tracking your basal body temperature will give you insight into whether and when you ovulated. At this time, you should also feel your cervix at a lower position than during ovulation, and it should be firmer, with sticky instead of slippery mucus.

If you are hitting all these marks after your expected ovulation date (elevated body temperature, high and firm cervix, sticky mucus), you can feel pretty confident that you ovulated. And if it is a healthy luteal phase, your cervical indicators and temperature should stay in this same place for about eleven to fourteen days. Any luteal phase shorter than that can be a sign of a luteal-phase deficiency, which means that your body isn't releasing as much progesterone (or isn't releasing progesterone for as long) as it's supposed to. If this happens to you more than occasionally, it may be worth going to see your health-care provider to find out if you have a condition that is contributing to chronic luteal-phase deficiency or whether your body is suppressing ovulation.

If you want to test at home whether you are producing sufficient levels of progesterone, you can get a test like Proov (which measures progesterone) or the Mira Hormone Monitor (which measures progesterone as well as other fertility hormones). Tests like these detect levels of the progesterone metabolite PdG in urine, which correlates almost perfectly with levels of progesterone in the blood, making it a great way to have a peek at your progesterone levels without having someone stick a needle in your arm. If you have PdG levels above 5 μg/mL throughout the implantation window (Days 20–24 in a twenty-eight-day cycle), it means you have ovulated and your body is releasing sufficient levels of progesterone to sustain implantation/

pregnancy *and* give you all the wonderful health benefits that progesterone offers (see chapter 9 if you need a reminder). If your levels are lower than this, it can indicate failure to ovulate or a luteal-phase deficiency.

Getting used to keeping track of your fertility status across the cycle can feel a little awkward at first. And when you're getting started, it's normal to lack confidence in what you think you're feeling or not feeling (Is this slippery? Or sticky? Or something else?). It can be really helpful to do things like use an at-home LH test to help validate things you think you're noticing in your daily fertility checks (*Ohhhhh, this is what my cervix feels like when it is soft*) or an at-home progesterone test to validate the things you think you're feeling when you're trying to confirm progesterone release (*Aha! I thought this was sticky!*). I used these tools when I was learning to understand my body too, and they helped me figure it all out. After that, though, they became unnecessary. I can tell when I'm having a healthy hormone-producing cycle and when I'm not with what I can only imagine is a pretty high degree of accuracy. Once you get well practiced in this, you will be able to do this too.

Things to Do Today to Improve Your Resilience to Hormonal Changes and Encourage Hormone Balance

In some ways, this section is redundant, but I thought it would be useful to end with a few closing notes to help summarize some of the main points we talked about here.

- The number one thing you can do to improve resilience to hormonal changes and promote healthy ovulation is to be in good health. The pillars of good health are eating foods that nourish the body, getting regular physical activity (steps taken while cooking count), getting enough sleep/having healthy circadian rhythms, managing stress, and having meaningful, supportive relationships with others. Maintaining these pillars of good health won't require you to spend a lot of money or turn your life upside down if you make gradual changes that improve your health. This month, you might incorporate into your routine chopping up vegetables at the beginning of the week to include in home-cooked meals throughout the week. Next month, you may add in taking walks outside in the morning to help set your circadian clock and get your body moving. And each week, see if you can find opportunities to connect with others by spending time with those you love, doing volunteer work, or attending community engagement events. When it comes to your health, you have to play the long game, so take your time developing habits that are easy for you to stick to over time.

- If any of the pillars of good health are deficient in your life, start taking stock of changes you can make to nudge yourself into better health. Take some time to jot down your ideas about ways you can support each of the pillars of good health (and make sure that the ideas you write down are things you are actually willing to do). After you write down your ideas, pick one or two of them that you are willing to commit to doing for at least three months. It takes three months for new practices to become habits, so it's important that you try to push through the three-month mark if you hope for a new habit to become something that you are able to do without thinking.
  - Eating foods that nourish the body
  - Getting regular physical activity
  - Getting enough sleep/having healthy circadian rhythms
  - Managing stress
  - Having or developing meaningful, supportive relationships with others

One of the things you can do to help increase the success of a new habit is to scaffold your newly developing habits onto your old ones. This is called habit stacking and it has been shown to increase the likelihood that a new habit will stick. For example, if you always spend thirty minutes having coffee in the morning, you can make this the time that you take your morning walk (if you follow my Instagram, you already know that I am a huge fan of the morning coffee walk—it's my favorite habit). Or if you usually catch up with your best friend from college on Sunday afternoons, you might add chopping up veggies into this routine. Stacking new habits onto old ones is a smart way to add positive changes into your life and increases the likelihood that they stick.

- If you have a lot of changes that need to be made to improve your health, don't let yourself get overwhelmed by trying to make too many changes at once. Our brains are creatures of habit and it's better to take smaller steps toward good health because they are more achievable. When we try to do too much, too soon, it can make us freak out because it feels disorienting. Your brain loves familiarity, and too much unfamiliarity at once (which is exactly what you end up with if you turn your whole life upside down) will make you crave the familiarity of your old ways of doing things. Make one positive change at a time so that you can increase the sticking power of your new, healthful habits.
- Track your cycles and make sure you are regularly ovulating. If you are not, consider adopting any or all of the practices mentioned in this chapter for promoting resilience to hormonal changes and regular ovulation. If you have already done everything mentioned in this chapter and continue to experience frequently disrupted ovulation or really bad PMS, consider talking to your health-care

provider about what's going on. There is a chance that there is an underlying health problem that needs to be addressed.

Although we are wired to feel different in the first half our cycles than we do in the second (the follicular phase is supposed to feel different from the luteal), taking active steps to promote the health of our bodies will make these changes less noticeable and jarring. It will also help support regular ovulation and hormonal balance, and will ensure that you get all the health benefits available from regular progesterone exposure.

CHAPTER 12

THE FUTURE IS SEX DIFFERENTIATED AND HORMONAL

The end of bikini science

As our time together draws to a close, I want you to join me in a thought experiment. Imagine a world where women's bodies are the standard for what is considered normal. Where all our institutions and practices are rooted in the experiences of women's bodies instead of those of men.

Imagine being taught from a young age about how your hormones cycle and how there are two halves to your whole. Imagine it being standard educational practice for all girls (and boys) to be given a foundational education in the way their bodies work. How would it change your life to know so much about your body that you never had to go to social media or buy a book like this one to help make sense of yourself? Can you imagine being so in tune with your body's hormonal changes that you would be able to identify what is going on with your primary sex hormones (Am I ovulating? Did I ovulate? Does my progesterone feel low?) without having to buy hormone tests or go to your doctor's office? Imagine having the seasons of your cycle be like second nature to you and being able to trust the wisdom of your body's changing needs instead of treating them with suspicion and resentment.

Now, I want you to imagine yourself at a gym where classes and equipment are divided based on cycle phase and pregnancy or menopausal status. On one side of the gym are heavy resistance machines and free weights for women in the follicular phase and perimenopausal/menopausal women,* while restorative exercise rooms are on the other side for women in the luteal phase or those who are pregnant. Imagine your personal trainer routinely asking about your cycle phase to guide you toward the most beneficial workout for your body.

Next, I want you to imagine that it is standard practice to have your cycle phase taken into account when making appointments with therapists and doctors. Imagine your therapist recognizing that your emotional needs shift throughout the month and setting up your treatments in a way that is sensitive to that. For example, if you were seeking extinction therapy (which is the treatment of choice for PTSD and phobias), you would have your sessions scheduled in the follicular phase, when research finds it to be most effective. Or if you were being counseled to help break a cycle of addiction, you'd be encouraged to begin your recovery in the luteal phase, when you're less likely to experience cravings. Imagine being given medication that you knew had been tested on female bodies and was dosed according to your hormonal changes rather than being given a one-size-fits-all treatment that was tested on men.

And this is only the beginning.

Imagine being in a world where teen girls are taught about their changing energy levels, nutritional needs, and caloric requirements across their cycle. Imagine growing up without the body hatred that gets created when women are set up to fail with one-size-fits-all nutritional advice that leaves them hungry, craving unhealthy foods, and feeling like failures. What would it feel like to see your body as a repository of inherited wisdom to be listened to and trusted rather than an enemy whose needs should be ignored?

Picture a world where menstrual products are available in public

---

* In case you haven't heard, women in perimenopause and menopause really, really benefit from resistance training to offset the muscle loss that occurs as we age.

restrooms, free of charge, like toilet paper. Where young girls in need don't have to worry about how their families will pay for their menstrual products over school breaks when they can't get them from the school nurse. Think about pregnancy, postpartum, lactation, and menopause support being considered an essential part of health care and the workplace. Where the support that women need during each of these phases is baked into what is considered standard care and practice.

Envision a world where sexual desire, moods, and even immune function are understood as cyclical processes. Where every major decision and challenge is considered incomplete until it has been viewed through the distinct influences of estrogen and progesterone. In this world, everyone would know and understand the optimal times for women to learn, have surgeries, get vaccinations—and both men and women would receive health care that respected the different ways that disease and treatments can affect their bodies.

Although such a world may seem a distant, airy-fairy fantasy, it doesn't need to be. It just feels that way because it is so far removed from what the world looks like now. The world as we know it was created for men and male bodies. Although I don't think the world was designed the way it was to intentionally exclude women, it has nonetheless harmed us. Because what works for male bodies doesn't always work for ours. What's good for the gander isn't necessarily good for the goose. Many of us feel hungry, exhausted, and angry at our bodies for not doing what we think they are supposed to do in the luteal phase because the world wasn't designed for women with cycles.

Making the world better suited for women's bodies means that we are going to need to change the way we think about sex and hormones. We need to acknowledge that they matter, sometimes deeply, for how our bodies respond to everything from emotional experiences and the relationships we have to the food we eat and the medicine we take. And though it might not feel like that big a revelation to acknowledge that sex and hormones matter and need to be accounted for in how we come to understand ourselves and those around us, it will require a fundamental shift in the assumptions that currently guide research practice in brain, behavioral, and clinical science.

So, let's get to it. First, we'll talk about how science needs to change so that clinical practice can serve men's and women's bodies equally. Then we'll talk about what each of us can do today to improve our ability to understand ourselves and advocate for the care we need.

The End of Bikini Science

When we began our time together in this book, we talked about the fact that the unique needs of women and female bodies are ignored in fields ranging from medicine and law to automobile design. We talked about how laws, drugs, and car safety features are created using male bodies and brains as the standard for what it looks like to be human, and how, because of this, there is much about our world that isn't well suited for women. We have cars that can't protect us, laws that don't safeguard our interests, and drugs that make us feel worse rather than better because the guiding assumption is that human = male.

The assumption that human = male creates a problem for everything about women that makes them different from men. And these differences often extend far deeper than the easy-to-see differences in our reproductive organs and sex hormones. These differences are *everywhere*. Creating a version of the world where science, medicine, innovation, and law actually serve the interests of men *and* women will require that we fundamentally change our assumptions about the nature of biological sex differences and hormonal changes across the cycle. We need to understand that our desire to ignore or minimize these differences in the name of convenience or fear of political fallout (which I will speak to) harms women. We will never have truly comprehensive care for those with female bodies until we recognize that biological sex matters deeply when it comes to all things health.

Unfortunately, we're nowhere close to this. Despite increased attention and funding being directed toward issues in women's health, the prevailing paradigm in science and medicine is still one that assumes women's health is synonymous with gynecology. This means that the funds currently being directed toward addressing the female health gap are going toward understanding conditions that affect female reproductive organs, but not much else. While this still benefits women—I think we can all agree it's high time we better understood things like endometriosis, PCOS, postpartum depression, and the menopausal transition—these sorts of issues represent only a tiny fraction of what women's health actually is. Women's health is about the health of women. And the health of women is something that extends throughout our entire bodies. It's cardiovascular care, brain health, cancer prevention, mental health care, immunology, and everything else that our bodies do. If the body in question is female, it is a women's health issue. It is only when we get really comfortable with this idea—and the fact that it will require rewriting some of the existing rules for doing science—that we will be able to create a world that is better suited to how women's bodies work. And when we do this, it will improve the state of health care for both women and men.

Currently, as science is practiced, sex is not something many researchers want to have to deal with. I can't tell you how commonplace it is for researchers to stick their findings in the file drawer (which is what we call it when we have research results we don't publish) because they can't account for the messiness in the data created by the inclusion of both males and females in their research. They don't know what to make of it—and because the prevailing paradigm in science is one that assumes a lack of sex differentiation, there is no basis for them to explain their results.

I was recently in a research talk by a colleague who found that a specific dietary intervention given to rodents to help prevent brain changes known to predict Alzheimer's disease had opposite effects on males and females. Rather than embrace the possibility that male Alzheimer's disease and female Alzheimer's disease may be two distinct diseases with different etiologies, symptoms, and developmental pathways (which, by the way, is the view that I am becoming increasingly convinced is true), my colleague concluded that their intervention "didn't work." And this was their conclusion despite the fact that it *did* work in 50 percent of their sample.

This happens more frequently than you might think in biomedical research that includes both males and females. When males and females don't respond the same way to a treatment or intervention (which they rarely do), many times the results either don't get published or the researchers try to minimize the differences between the sexes so that they can publish their "messy"[*] results without creating waves in the status quo or having to come up with an explanation for the differences. There is a reluctance for researchers to stick their necks out there and say what so many have long suspected, but few have been willing to say:[†] males and females are different. And we may be different enough that it requires revising our basic assumptions about the impact of biological sex on research outcomes.

This is exactly what I am advocating we need to do. In my view, if we are to have any hope at all of actually improving the state of health and wellness care for women (and men! I care about them too!), science needs a do-over.[‡] We need to change the working assumptions that scientists use when designing research studies so that women can be studied and understood as being distinct from men in

---

[*] Messy in science is when you have results that don't fit neatly into whatever theoretical narrative you have created to explain them.

[†] There are some wonderful exceptions to this rule, including researchers doing some really exciting work looking at things like sex differences in the mechanisms that cause and prevent cancer, sex differences in the ways that our cells respond to DNA damage, and the molecular basis of sex-specific therapeutic responses to various types of medical treatment. Wonderful scientists like Catherine Woolley and others have been presenting high-quality science demonstrating that key molecular processes in the brain (and they're "key" because they affect everything) differ between the sexes in important ways.

[‡] Just like you used to do when you were a kid playing a game with friends. If you made a mistake, you would often ask for a do-over. This would allow you to hit the reset button, forget what happened before, and try again.

ways that extend beyond the obvious. The bikini science approach to biomedical research needs to become a thing of the past.

The scientific do-over I am advocating for would require adopting the following two assumptions in the development of new biomedical research:

- **Starting assumption number 1: Biological sex matters and the existence of sex differences should be assumed until proven otherwise.** Male and female subjects need to be tested in equal and high-enough numbers to have sufficient statistical power* to test for sex differences. If a researcher wants to exclude sex as a variable in their research and simply lump male and female subjects together in their research design, it is up to them to first convincingly demonstrate that biological sex doesn't matter by either (a) using high-quality data with sufficient statistical power to test for sex differences on the measured trait and demonstrate that there aren't any, or (b) citing other studies that have convincingly demonstrated that the sexes don't differ on the measured dimension using high-quality data and sufficiently powered statistical tests.

    Adopting this as a starting assumption will also require that journal editors and research panel reviewers at funding agencies get comfortable with sex differentiation and be patient with scientists as they scramble to figure out what these differences mean. There will be a period of time where people will be reporting sex differentiation

---

* This means that there are enough males and females in a sample to be able to find evidence of sex differentiation in a trait if such differentiation exists. And (believe it or not) this is *not* a requirement for research right now. Although federally funded health research must include males and females, it does not require that researchers have enough of each sex in their sample to find sex differences if such differences exist *nor* does it require that researchers actually look for differences. It honestly makes no f*cking sense at all.

that they have only speculative explanations for, and we all need to accept this as part of the process to move things forward. Editors and funders need to get comfortable with publishing and funding things with only tentative answers about the cause of sex differentiation.

Coming to terms with the fact that many diseases and responses to treatments may be sex differentiated will also require scientists and researchers to develop policies or rules of thumb about how to handle sex-differentiated outcomes. Should a researcher studying a disease that seems to have a different developmental trajectory in males and females be required to study the disease in both sexes? Or if we feel it is too steep of an ask to have a single lab figure out the way things work in both sexes,[*] how can we ensure that equal attention is given to male and female disease pathways? These are important questions that need to be addressed as we move in this direction. They may be tricky to answer, but the benefit of muddling through them in the name of better science will be worth it.

- **Starting assumption number 2: Sex hormones and cycle phase matter and need to be studied rather than statistically controlled for.** When we begin to study women separately from men, it makes it possible for women to be tested *as* women. We can move away from the practice of

---

[*] Although you may have a knee-jerk "of course they should have to figure it out in both sexes" reaction, no one would expect someone who specializes in prostate cancer in men to have to also figure out uterine, endometrial, cervical, or ovarian cancer in women. Although this isn't the perfect analogy, if there is a disease process that operates differently in male and female bodies, studying them both would require understanding all the nuances of both male and female bodies. This may be something that is very feasible, or it may not be. It may be better for research labs to specialize in disease processes as they unfold in either male or female bodies, since specialization may allow for more nuanced insights. This is an important conversation to have if we are to adopt my recommendation that sex differences be assumed as the starting point in science.

statistically controlling for the effects of our sex hormones on outcomes and instead start measuring them. To this end, researchers should be required to test women and female subjects in each major phase* of the menstrual cycle to allow us to understand whether women's responses to experimental manipulations differ across the cycle. Here again, if researchers wish to lump all women together in their research design (i.e., not account for cycle phase), it is up to them to first convincingly demonstrate that cycle phase doesn't matter, either (a) with their own high-quality data that fails to find differences across the cycle or (b) by citing other studies that have convincingly demonstrated that cycle phase doesn't matter.

Adopting this assumption in research science—in addition to making it possible for the first time in history for women to be studied as women—will also create a needed paradigm shift around the relative importance of progesterone. Although much of the research on women's sex hormones to date has focused exclusively on estrogen, changing our assumptions about the importance of each of our hormonal states emphasizes the fact that progesterone matters too. Because it does. Changing this assumption would make it necessary for researchers examining the role of female sex hormones on outcomes like sexual function, hot flashes, autoimmune disease, or the development of Alzheimer's disease to look at the impact of both hormones. Currently, there is a myopic focus on estrogen for outcomes like these, despite there being every reason

---

* In a perfect world, we would get more granular yet and look at the menstrual/early follicular phase, ovulatory phase, early luteal phase, and late luteal phase, but that, at least for now, would be cost-, time-, and sanity-prohibitive. It is hard enough to systematically account for two phases in research. Starting with the two major phases will get us into a position where we know how women's bodies respond in the season of each of our primary sex hormones. This alone will put us into a much stronger position to care for women's health.

to suspect that progesterone may also be at play. I am confident that there is a lot that we can learn about women's health and psychological functioning when we take off the estrogen blinders and correct the current hormonal imbalance in research.

If this is all we do to change the practice of science, it will be a huge step in the right direction. It would allow us to understand so much more about women than what we do currently. It would give women a female-specific view of what is normal for them. It would allow us to better understand disease progression in both women and men, since lumping them together slows progress by blurring the real picture of what's happening in each sex. It would also allow physicians to provide women with better treatment. They would be able to better address patient concerns, such as "Why do I feel this way at this time, but not at the other?" or "Why do I have this mysterious symptom?" because women will be studied and understood as women.

Women are often frustrated by their health care and the inability of their doctors to provide them with answers for the ways they feel. This is understandable given the frequency with which women are misdiagnosed, unable to be diagnosed, or made to feel that their symptoms are all in their head. But medicine can only be as good as the science that informs its practice. And science has failed women. When science takes sex and hormones seriously, medical practice will follow. Most doctors I know *want* to serve the needs of their female patients but feel helpless at the lack of information available on the things women care about. They don't have a full picture of what health and disorder actually look like in women since research has historically been done on men. I am convinced that when science does better, medicine will do better. Bikini medicine will only die when we demand that the research establishment puts an end to bikini science.

Emphasizing the importance of biological sex and hormonal changes in science and medicine can feel scary in a political landscape that can feel hostile to women. And a lot of us feel that way right now. Women have been dealt some serious blows to our rights in recent years that have left many of us wondering what will be taken away next. I share these concerns with you. The idea of living in a world where my daughter will have fewer rights and less sovereignty over her body than I have had over mine is crushing. It can be really tempting to want to downplay the things about us that make us different from men because, if we're not that different from men, maybe there is nothing else that can be taken from us.

But this isn't the solution to our current political climate. Acknowledging the importance of biological sex does not in any way preclude our deservedness of rights. It also does not minimize the importance of gender. Denying the fact that female bodies are different from male bodies—in addition to being an ineffective strategy for protecting our freedoms (sexist a**holes will find an excuse for their behavior, regardless of what we do)—is bad for us. In addition to providing researchers with a far-too-convenient excuse to exclude women from research (or to equate women's health with gynecology), it reinforces the prevailing cultural assumption that male = normal and therefore female = problematic.

The fact is, male = normal is true for males. And female = normal is true for females. And there is no one way of being that is better than the other because they are each exactly what they are supposed to be based on their different evolutionary paths. Normal for males is characterized by the presence of one primary hormone that declines slowly with age (which is the same pattern we see for virtually all sexually reproducing organisms whose only contribution to reproduction is sex). Normal for females is characterized by two primary sex hormones that cycle (which is what is necessary for sexually reproducing organisms whose contributions to reproduction include both sex and pregnancy). The belief that male = normal is nothing more than an artifact of the fact that men were studied first and, because of that, are the ones whose physiology was used to create our collective rough draft of what it means to be human.

It's time to make the necessary revisions.

Our ability to create for our daughters the sort of world that serves men's and women's needs equally will require coming to terms with the fact that biological sex and hormones matter in how people think, feel, and experience the world. It will require that we recognize a need for creating health and practice standards that are sex- and cycle-phase-specific. We should know what "normal" looks like for men and what "normal" looks like for women. And we should be smart and respectful enough of the limitations of "normal" to understand that these guidelines are not prescriptive and won't account for everyone's experiences in the world. Women's health is about the health of women. And it's only when we move beyond our outdated assumptions about sex and hormones that we can truly advance the state of knowledge about women's bodies in sickness and in health. It is my hope that this book will move us one step closer to making this a reality.

The Future and Beyond: Pregnancy, Postpartum, Perimenopause, and Menopause

As science begins to progress in a way that demands that women be studied as women, the next steps will necessarily involve developing a greater understanding of women's brains and bodies as they transition through other hormonal changes that transcend the cycle. Puberty, pregnancy, postpartum, perimenopause, and menopause are all periods of huge hormonal transition for women and need to be understood both as states (e.g., what does perimenopause look like?) as well as conditions in which women's responses to treatments of all sorts are likely to vary.

Thankfully, there is some really beautiful work being done by research labs such as those headed by Dr. Claudia Barth, Dr. Emily Jacobs, Dr. Lisa Mosconi, Dr. Jerilynn Prior, and others who are looking at changes in the brain and elsewhere in the body during pregnancy, postpartum, and menopause. Their research finds that women's brains and bodies really are dynamic processes that constantly evolve in response to our changing hormonal states. There is so much value to women in understanding what they are going through in these hormonally dynamic states, and women are hungry to know what is happening and to be given a mirror to reflect who they are becoming at these times.

But there is so much more that needs to be done. We know very little about whether different types of medical and psychological interventions—ranging from the use of medication to the use of something like cognitive behavioral therapy—differ depending on pregnancy, postpartum, and menopausal status. These questions are important and have implications for virtually all women at various points in their life. Moving beyond the overly simplistic, one-size-fits-all view of what it means to be human will mean diving more deeply into the different stages of womanhood to provide women with appropriate guidelines that work for their bodies in those states. It is my hope that the future of science will be a future that continues to push the existing limitations on what is known about women by expanding to study women as women, in all of our different manifestations across our lifetime.

To Thine Own Cycle Be True

Although we are not yet in a place where we know enough about the impact of women's cycling hormones to create a world that is truly cut out to address women's changing needs, there are things that each of us can do today to help bring our own reality closer to that world.

The first is that we can track our cycles. I know that I have repeated this about a hundred times, but you will gain so much from learning how you change across the cycle. Being attuned to your body's changing needs is the first step in advocating for yourself with your doctor and really understanding yourself. Use the cycle-tracking resources I have provided for you in appendix A (or create your own!) to track your mood, energy levels, sexual desire, physical symptoms, medication side effects, hunger, food cravings, and whatever else it is about yourself that you want to understand. Reading books like this one and educating yourself about your hormones are great first steps toward developing body literacy, but nothing (nothing!) can replace the huge depth of self-understanding that you can get from simply tracking your own cycle over time.

Tracking your cycle and learning about your unique response to your hormonal changes will give you insight about yourself that you can't get from a doctor, a book, or conversations with your girlfriends. Because no two of us are exactly alike, and the way your body responds to hormonal changes across the cycle may be different from the way most other people's bodies respond. Our brains differ from one another, our hormone levels differ from one another, the density of our hormone receptors differ from one another, the way we metabolize our hormones differs from one another, the ins and outs of our body's other endocrine (hormone) systems differ from one another, our patterns of gene expression differ from one another . . . we're just all a little different. And because of this—no matter what it is you're talking about—there will always be differences and there will always be outliers. This means that, for some of us, the usual set of rules will not apply.

For example, with mood, although most women exhibit a pattern in which progesterone is linked with low-level melancholy and pessimism/anxiety (all of those preparing-for-pregnancy-danger-sensitized-brain changes we talked about in chapter 5), we don't see this pattern in everyone. Some women don't experience many changes at all, some women's changes are exaggeratedly terrible, and for others they're totally upside down. In one study, for example, researchers had 213 naturally cycling female college students each keep a mood diary over two cycles. Researchers then mapped women's daily moods onto their menstrual data to look at changes in how women felt based on cycle phase. What they found was that, although most women (61 percent) exhibited a classic PMS-like pattern (with mood worsening in the luteal phase compared to the follicular), some women reported no cyclical changes in mood at all (26 percent), and some women demonstrated a pattern of worsening mood near ovulation (13 percent) when most research finds that women feel *good*.

See why it is so important to know your own body? Women are

routinely found to vary in how they respond to the hormonal changes across the cycle. Although each of us is a little different, research finds most women are remarkably consistent in their own patterns. For example, if you are someone who feels emotionally worse during the luteal phase, this is likely to be fairly consistently true of you from cycle to cycle. And if you are someone who feels relatively stable in your mood across the cycle, this is likely to be consistently true too.

Understanding whether your hormonal changes affect how you feel—and if they do, how—can be a total game changer in your relationship with yourself and others. It can also help us better communicate with our health-care providers to make sure we get the care we need. Women who experience depressed mood in the luteal phase are at a greater risk of developing mood disorders after giving birth (postpartum depression) and during the perimenopausal transition. And my guess is that this is just the tip of the iceberg. Knowing that your _____ [sex drive, appetite, asthma, eating disorder, fill in the blank with whatever it is for you] is sensitive to hormonal changes across the cycle will likely increase the risk of having issues with your _____ [fill in the blank with the same word] postpartum and in perimenopause. Knowing this and being able to communicate about it with your caregiver may help ensure you get the care you need (and at a time when you need it most).

Keeping track of changes in how you feel across the cycle will also allow you to better care for yourself and advocate for yourself in relationships. If you notice that you are consistently hungrier in the luteal phase, you can consider increasing your calorie intake. If you have changing sexual desire, you can talk to your partner. If you feel like you're spinning your wheels at the gym in the luteal phase, you can try shifting up your routine to be more in tune with what's going on hormonally . . . the list of adjustments we can make to improve the quality of our lives is endless. Knowing how your body responds to your hormonal changes will put you in the driver's seat when it comes to taking control of your mental and physical health.

We are just getting warmed up in terms of what we know about how women's hormonal changes across the cycle and lifespan affect who we are and help define our lives. And each of us can be a part of that growing awareness by monitoring ourselves and helping create a world designed for women.

Closing Thoughts

I want to close this book by having you think back to our thought experiment about a world created for women's bodies. Where women are studied and understood as women and the world is laid out in a way that supports our bodies' needs instead of fighting against them. I now want you to think of the ways that you can help create this world for yourself. What steps can you take to make your life better suited to the needs of your body? How can you help your friends, daughters, and others do the same?

For too long, women have been made to feel like inferior versions of men and our hormonal changes treated as a form of weakness or pathology—a nuisance variable to be controlled for in research and ignored by medicine. The result is that we have only been told half of our story. For some of us, this has created PMS and the development of unpleasant symptoms arising from trying to get our bodies to conform to one-size-fits-all rules. For others, it has created unnecessary worry about what's wrong with us when our sexual desire or physical symptoms change across the cycle. And for others still, it has completely destroyed our relationship with ourselves, creating a belief that our body is the enemy when it fights back in response to our failure to give it what it needs in the season of progesterone.

It is time for this to end.

We deserve to live in a world where our bodies are understood in the season of both of our primary sex hormones, and where the guidance we are given to help us understand who we are and what our bodies need honors this cyclicity. This will require nothing short of a complete do-over in the way that women are treated in science and medicine. And for some of us, it will require reimagining our relationship with ourselves. When we listen to the changing needs of our body as wisdom instead of pathology—and recognize that our needs are not one size fits all—we can finally walk away from the story of our body as the enemy. Let's be part of the generation that changes the narrative about women's hormones and redefines women's health to be about the health of women. Together, we can redefine "normal" and usher in an era of greater self-understanding for women, one cycle at a time.

APPENDIX A

Below is where you can download a free cycle-tracking diary from Dr. Jerilynn Prior, who is a total rock star in the world of women's reproductive health. I also encourage you to check out her other resources. She is an absolute bad*ss scientist and advocate for the importance of progesterone. She is who I want to be when I grow up.

https://www.cemcor.ca/resources/daily-menstrual-cycle-diary

If you are looking for a more simplified guide, you can also download a free cycle-tracking guide on my website. Go to sarahehill.com/cycle-tracker to download either a digital or printable guide to help you track your experiences across the cycle.

Things to Remember

- The first day of your cycle (Cycle Day 1) is the first day of bleeding on your period.
- If you are measuring body temperature, do it first thing in the morning as soon as you wake up.

How to Identify Ovulation and Cycle Phase Using the Back-Counting Method

- From Day 1 of your second cycle, count back fourteen days. These fourteen days were likely the luteal phase in your last cycle.
  - Confirm your luteal phase using your recorded body temperature data. If your temperature was elevated relative to what it was in the earlier part of your cycle, you can feel more confident that (a) you ovulated, and (b) you were in your luteal phase.
- Ovulation likely occurred the day prior to the start of your luteal phase.
  - Confirm ovulation by referencing your cervical mucus data (it will have been slippery and clear, like egg whites).
  - Confirm ovulation by temperature data (our body temperature dips right near ovulation).
    - ~ Note that I can't always capture this temperature dip using wearable tech, even when I have successfully ovulated. Just FYI in case you run into that problem too.
- All the days prior to ovulation are your follicular phase, with the five-ish days prior to ovulation (and the day of ovulation itself) being your fertile window.

Tips and Tricks for Measuring Your Moods, Sexual Desire, Etc., Across the Cycle

- Rate how you are feeling at the same time every day. I like doing end of day since it's hard to know how we feel on a given day as soon as we wake up. However, you can do it right when you wake up if that's easier for you. Just reflect on the prior day.

- Don't overthink it. This is what kills most women's cycle tracking. Don't give up because you're not sure if you're remembering things correctly. Just do your best and you will get valuable data. I promise.
- If the cycle trackers recommended here overwhelm you, consider making your own simplified version that captures the things you are most interested in measuring.

Other Recommendations

- I use wearable tech to log my body temperature (and everything else). I love the Oura Ring and the Apple Watch. I have friends who love the WHOOP band. Some people don't like wearables because the data might not be as precise as what you might get if you measured your own temperature every day, but for me, the pluses far outweigh the minuses. I am really bad at remembering to measure my BBT in the morning, so wearable tech has allowed me to consistently track my temps without having to think about it too much.
- 28 is an app that tracks your cycle using temperature inputs from your Apple Watch or using your own manual cycle or temperature inputs. It also allows you to track your moods, sexual desire, energy levels, and a whole bunch of other stuff as it changes across the cycle. Of all the cycle trackers, I like it the best. The big reason I like it the best is because I helped contribute to its design. We have designed it in a way that allows you to see quantifiable changes in how you are feeling at different points in your cycle and also to see improvements in or worsening of symptoms over time. But I also love it because it provides daily recipes and workouts that are tailored for each cycle phase, making it simple to care for ourselves in a way that accounts for our cyclicity.

APPENDIX B

Here are some cookbooks and cooking websites that I love. Please note that (a) I have no financial relationships with any of these people or companies, and (b) there are probably a number of others out there that are just as good that I don't know about. These are just the ones that I use.

Also note that many of these have primarily or exclusively plant-based recipes. Feel free to add animal protein to any of the recipes. Using plant-based recipes as a starting point can help ensure you are getting a lot of flavor and health benefits from plants before adding animal protein.

Love Real Food, **Kathryne Taylor**
Kathryne has recipes online too, at cookieandkate.com.

The Oh She Glows Cookbook, **Angela Liddon**
Angela has recipes online too, at ohsheglows.com/recipe-categories.

Love and Lemons: Simple Feel Good Food, **Jeanine Donofrio**
Jeanine also has other cookbooks, but this is the one I use the most. She has recipes online too, at loveandlemons.com.

The Minimalist Baker

https://minimalistbaker.com/recipe-index/

The 28 Wellness App

This app has cycle-phase-inspired recipes that are delicious and ensure that you get enough to eat in the luteal phase. It also includes grocery lists, which I find super helpful. Its breakfast recipes are constantly in the rotation at my house because everyone likes them (even those members of my household without cycles).

***Everyday Food: Great Food Fast: 250 Recipes for Easy, Delicious Meals All Year Long: A Cookbook,* From the Kitchens of Martha Stewart Living**

I love this cookbook because everything has a relatively few number of ingredients and can be made pretty quickly.

APPENDIX C

Cycle-Supporting Products I Love

I get asked a lot about the products I love that help support my cycle. Here are some of the ones I use. Note that I am not being paid to promote these products. They are all products I actually use. If you go to the "Products I Love" page on my website, you will find discount codes to give you a percentage off your purchase.

For supplements, I love the ones from BIOptimizers. Here are the ones I take:

- Magnesium Breakthrough. I love this magnesium because it contains seven different types of magnesium to support health. I felt the difference immediately in my sleep when I switched to this brand and you will too. Make sure you take it at bedtime because it really does chill you out and make you sleepy.
- Sleep Breakthrough. I also love this product and take it when I am keyed up and need extra help dialing things down before bedtime. It feels a little like taking melatonin, but is melatonin-free, so it doesn't lower testosterone (yes, melatonin is antagonistic to testosterone).

For tracking my cycle and getting recipes and workouts to support my cycle, I love 28 Wellness's cycle-based wellness app. In the spirit of full transparency, note that I am a science adviser for 28. But I want to emphasize that I am an adviser for this company because I believe in the product, not because of a financial incentive. The results of our recent research with 28 found that using the exercise and nutrition guidance in the app led to improved fitness and wellness outcomes for women, making me even more confident that it works.

If you want to test your progesterone at home or want to do a full hormone work-up, the products I love are from Proov. They are inexpensive, easy to use, and the founder is a science bad*ss who is trying to make the world a better place for women.

I wear nontoxic workout wear from MATE the Label. Most yoga pants have endocrine-disrupting chemicals in them, but these do not. They are also flattering and comfy (luteal-phase-approved comfort!).

APPENDIX D

Other Great Hormone Books and an Initiation to Learn More

Period Help

- *Period Repair Manual*, Lara Briden
- *The Fifth Vital Sign*, Lisa Hendrickson-Jack
- *Fix Your Period*, Nicole Jardim

Perimenopause/Menopause Help

- *Hormone Repair Manual*, Lara Briden
- *The Upgrade*, Louann Brizendine, MD
- *Perimenopause Power*, Maisie Hill
- *The Menopause Brain*, Lisa Mosconi, PhD

Hormone Help

- *The Hormone Cure*, Sara Gottfried, MD
- *The Hormone Balance Bible*, Shawn Tassone, MD, PhD
- *Hormone Intelligence*, Aviva Romm, MD

Learning About Your Cycle/Cycle-Based Wellness

- *The Hormone Reset Diet*, Sara Gottfried, MD
- *Period Power*, Maisie Hill

- *In the Flo*, Alisa Vitti
- *Woman Code*, Alisa Vitti

Female Brain/Brain Support

- *The Female Brain*, Louann Brizendine, MD
- *The XX Brain*, Lisa Mosconi, PhD

Hormonal Birth Control

- *Beyond the Pill*, Dr. Jolene Brighten
- *This Is Your Brain on Birth Control*, Sarah E. Hill, PhD (look, even the president votes for himself)

You can also learn more by following me on social media (@sarahehillphd on all social media handles) and visiting my webpage at sarahehill.com. On my website, I have links to research papers as well as video links and downloads to learn from me.

ACKNOWLEDGMENTS

I owe a huge thank-you to my amazing family for supporting me during this process. June and James: You are my life's masterpiece and the inspiration behind everything I do. Mom: Thank you for always being the first reader of every chapter I have ever written and always being my number-one fan; I don't know what I would do without you. Jim: You have been my soft place to land during this writing process and in life; you make me want to be better, always.

I want to thank the following people for offering me feedback and assistance with various stages of this book: Ann Beardsley, Sarah Angle, Lara Briden, Kristina Durante, Jerilynn Prior, Gabby Reece: Thank you all for helping me talk through my chapters or answering my content questions with your expertise. Madison Brown: Thank you for being an absolute star with the researching and reference generating needed to make this book happen. Katja Cunningham: Thank you for your amazing illustrations. Thank you also to everyone who has done the important research that I talk about in this book. You are doing a huge service to women with your tireless efforts, and I hope you'll forgive me if I've messed up any of the details or oversimplified things beyond what you consider to be in good taste. I look forward to continuing to learn from all the things you do.

Many friends, colleagues, collaborators, mentors, and students have helped me in other ways, whether it has been in teaching me new things, collaborating with me on research, helping me brainstorm ideas, or just being willing to put up with the fact that I have been distracted and not as available as I would like to be. In no particular order other than alphabetical, I'd like to thank Olivia Baldner, Jim Beardsley, Hannah Bradshaw, Jolene Brighten, Melissa Brillhart, Louann Brizendine, David Buss, Stephen Butler, Max Butterfield, Tracy Centanni, Talia Chachkes, Catherine Coleman, Merrell Davis, Danielle DelPriore, Jeff Gassen, Greg Eickholt, James Eickholt, June Eickholt, Abby Epstein, Matthew Espinosa, Suzanne Gilberg-Lenz, Jim Griffin, Savannah Hastings, Jim Hill, Joe Horn, Emily Jacobs, Nicole Jardim, Christina Kostaralis, Ricki Lake, Summer Mengelkoch, Shardi Nahavandi, Victoria Orozco, Jerilynn Prior, Randi Proffitt, Marjorie Prokosch, Kern Reeve, Christopher Rodeheffer, Mariza Snyder, Ingrid Tulloch, Wendy Williams, Ruby Winocur, Michael Winterdahl, Misty Womack, and the team at 28 Wellness.

To my amazing readers, students, and followers: I hope you have as much fun learning as I have teaching you all.

Lastly, I owe a huge thank you to my incredible agent, Lindsay Edgecombe, and my equally incredible editor, Sarah Pelz. I can't thank you all enough for your support and for sharing my vision for this book. Thank you also to all the folks at Harvest and LGR who have worked behind the scenes to make all this possible.

Thank you, thank you, thank you.

NOTES

Chapter 1: Why Do We All Have PMS?

4   *researchers looked at data:* Pierson, E., Althoff, T., Thomas, D., Hillard, P., & Leskovec, J. (2021). Daily, weekly, seasonal and menstrual cycles in women's mood, behaviour and vital signs. *Nature Human Behaviour, 5*(6), 716–25.

6   *experience low self-esteem:* Tempel, R. (2001). PMS in the workplace: An occupational health nurse's guide to premenstrual syndrome. *AAOHN Journal, 49*(2), 72–78.

6   *comparable to major depressive disorder:* Halbreich, U., Borenstein, J., Pearlstein, T., & Kahn, L. S. (2003). The prevalence, impairment, impact, and burden of premenstrual dysphoric disorder (PMS/PMDD). *Psychoneuroendocrinology, 28*(Suppl 3), 1–23.

6   *The risk of suicidality:* Prasad, D., Wollenhaupt-Aguiar, B., Kidd, K. N., de Azevedo Cardoso, T., & Frey, B. N. (2021). Suicidal risk in women with premenstrual syndrome and premenstrual dysphoric disorder: A systematic review and meta-analysis. *Journal of Women's Health (Larchmont), 30*(12), 1693–707.

6   *exposure to toxic chemicals has gone up:* Clatici, V. G., Voicu, C., Voaides, C., Roseanu, A., Icriverzi, M., & Jurcoane, S. (2018). Diseases of civilization—cancer, diabetes, obesity and acne—the implication of milk, IGF-1 and mTORC1. *Maedica (Bucur), 13*(4), 273–81.

7   *causes rats and mice:* Olsson, M., Ho, H.-P., Annerbrink, K., Melchior, L. K., Hedner, J., & Eriksson, E. (2003). Association between estrus cycle-related changes in respiration and estrus cycle-related aggression in outbred female wistar rats. *Neuropsychopharmacology, 28*(4), 704–10; Swanson, H. H., van de Poll, N. E., & van Pelt, J. (1982). Influence of the estrous cycle on heterosexual aggression in two strains of rats (S3 and WEzob). *Hormones and Behavior, 16*(4), 395–403.

7   *observed in vervet monkeys:* Rapkin, A. J., Pollack, D. B., Raleigh, M. J., Stone, B., & McGuire, M. T. (1995). Menstrual cycle and social behavior in vervet monkeys. *Psychoneuroendocrinology, 20*(3), 289–97.

7   *and even dairy cows:* Castellanos, F., Orihuela, A., & Galina, C. (1992). Aggressive behaviour in oestrus and dioestrus dairy cows and heifers. *Veterinary Record, 131,* 515–15.

9   *They. Affect. Everything:* Barth, C., Villringer, A., & Sacher, J. (2015). Sex hormones affect neurotransmitters and shape the adult female brain during hormonal transition periods [Review]. *Frontiers in Neuroscience, 9;* Brinton, R. D., Thompson, R. F., Foy, M. R., Baudry, M., Wang, J., Finch, C. E., Morgan, T. E., Pike, C. J., Mack, W. J., Stanczyk, F. Z., & Nilsen, J. (2008). Progesterone receptors: Form and function in brain. *Frontiers in Neuroendocrinology, 29*(2), 313–39.

Chapter 2: Understanding Your Cycle

14 *sexual desire, sexual function:* Nguyen, V., Leonard, A., and Heieh, T.-C., Testosterone and sexual desire: A review of the evidence. (2022). *Androgens: Clinical Research and Therapeutics, 3*(1), 85–90.

14 *lifetime sexual partners:* Pollet, T. V., van der Meij, L., Cobey, K. D., & Buunk, A. P. (2011). Testosterone levels and their associations with lifetime number of opposite sex partners and remarriage in a large sample of American elderly men and women. *Hormones and Behavior, 60*(1), 72–77.

14 *attracting serious dating partners:* Gettler, L. T., McDade, T. W., Feranil, A. B., & Kuzawa, C. W. (2011). Longitudinal evidence that fatherhood decreases testosterone in human males. *Proceedings of the National Academy of Sciences, 108*(39), 16194–99.

14 *extra-pair or casual sexual partners:* Peters, M., Simmons, L. W., & Rhodes, G. (2008). Testosterone is associated with mating success but not attractiveness or masculinity in human males. *Animal Behaviour, 76*(2), 297–303.

14 *clinicians regularly report:* Defreyne, J., Elaut, E., Kreukels, B., Fisher, A. D., Castellini, G., Staphorsius, A., Den Heijer, M., Heylens, G., & T'Sjoen, G. (2020). Sexual desire changes in transgender individuals upon initiation of hormone treatment: Results from the longitudinal European network for the investigation of gender incongruence. *Journal of Sexual Medicine, 17*(4), 812–25.

15 *you can turn sexual behavior:* Mazzola, C. R., & Mulhall, J. P. (2012). Impact of androgen deprivation therapy on sexual function. *Asian Journal of Andrology, 14*(2), 198–203.

15 *status, power, and other resources:* Dreher, J. C., Dunne, S., Pazderska, A., Frodl, T., Nolan, J. J., & O'Doherty, J. P. (2016). Testosterone causes both prosocial and antisocial status-enhancing behaviors in human males. *Proceedings of*

the National Academy of Science USA, 113(41), 11633–38; Eisenegger, C., Haushofer, J., & Fehr, E. (2011). The role of testosterone in social interaction. *Trends in Cognitive Science, 15*(6), 263–71.

15 **willingness to take risks:** White, R. E., Thornhill, S., & Hampson, E. (2006). Entrepreneurs and evolutionary biology: The relationship between testosterone and new venture creation. *Organizational Behavior and Human Decision Processes, 100*(1), 21–34.

15 **wealth-signaling luxury:** Nave, G., Nadler, A., Dubois, D., Zava, D., Camerer, C., & Plassmann, H. (2018). Single-dose testosterone administration increases men's preference for status goods. *Nature Communications, 9*(1), 2433.

15 **displays of generosity:** Nepomuceno, M. V., Saad, G., Stenstrom, E., Mendenhall, Z., & Iglesias, F. (2016). Testosterone & gift-giving: Mating confidence moderates the association between digit ratios (2D:4D and rel2) and erotic gift-giving. *Personality and Individual Differences, 91*, 27–30; Eisenegger, C., Naef, M., Snozzi, R., Heinrichs, M., & Fehr, E. (2010). Prejudice and truth about the effect of testosterone on human bargaining behaviour. *Nature, 463*(7279), 356–59.

15 **particularly toward partners:** Stanton, S. J. (2017). The role of testosterone and estrogen in consumer behavior and social & economic decision making: A review. *Hormones and Behavior, 92*, 155–63; Nepomuceno, M. V., Saad, G., Stenstrom, E., Mendenhall, Z., & Iglesias, F. (2016). Testosterone at your fingertips: Digit ratios (2D:4D and rel2) as predictors of courtship-related consumption intended to acquire and retain mates. *Journal of Consumer Psychology, 26*(2), 231–44.

15 **how sexy we feel:** Schleifenbaum, L., Driebe, J. C., Gerlach, T. M., Penke, L., & Arslan, R. C. (2021). Women feel more attractive before ovulation: Evidence from a large-scale online diary study. *Evolutionary Human Sciences, 3*, e47.

15 **our motivation for sex:** Roney, J. R., & Simmons, Z. L. (2013). Hormonal predictors of sexual motivation in natural menstrual cycles. *Hormones and Behavior, 63*(4), 636–45.

19 **the endometrium is open:** Harper, M. J. (1992). The implantation window. *Baillieres Clinical Obstetrics and Gynaecology, 6*(2), 351–71.

Chapter 3: How Ignoring Progesterone Created PMS

25 **researchers had 1,066:** Stanislaw, H., & and Rice, F. J. (1988). Correlation between sexual desire and menstrual cycle characteristics. *Archives of Sexual Behavior, 17*(6), 499–508.

25 **has since been replicated:** Arslan, R. C., Schilling, K. M., Gerlach, T. M., & and Penke, L. (2021). Using 26,000 diary entries to show ovulatory changes in sex-

ual desire and behavior. *Journal of Personality and Social Psychology, 121*(2), 410–31; Marcinkowska, U. M., Mijas, M., Koziara, K., Grebe, N. M., & Jasienska, G. (2021). Variation in sociosexuality across natural menstrual cycles: Associations with ovarian hormones and cycle phase. *Evolution and Human Behavior, 42*(1), 35–42.

26 **heterosexual women have more sex:** Wilcox, A. J., Baird, D. D., Dunson, D. B., McConnaughey, D. R., Kesner, J. S., & Weinberg, C. R. (2004). On the frequency of intercourse around ovulation: Evidence for biological influences. *Human Reproduction, 19*(7), 1539–43.

26 **Lesbian women have more sex:** Burleson, M. H., Trevathan, W. R., & Gregory, W. L. (2002). Sexual behavior in lesbian and heterosexual women: Relations with menstrual cycle phase and partner availability. *Psychoneuroendocrinology, 27*(4), 489–503.

26 **masturbation levels increase:** Harvey, S. M. (1987). Female sexual behavior: Fluctuations during the menstrual cycle. *Journal of Psychosomatic Research, 31*(1), 101–10; Jones, B. C., Hahn, A. C., Fisher, C. I., Wang, H., Kandrik, M., & DeBruine, L. M. (2018). General sexual desire, but not desire for uncommitted sexual relationships, tracks changes in women's hormonal status. *Psychoneuroendocrinology, 88*, 153–57.

26 **researchers had women come into:** Durante, K. M., Li, N. P., & Haselton, M. G. (2008). Changes in women's choice of dress across the ovulatory cycle: Naturalistic and laboratory task-based evidence. *Personality and Social Psychology Bulletin, 34*(11), 1451–60.

28 **make food seem less:** Richard, J. E., López-Ferreras, L., Anderberg, R. H., Olandersson, K., & Skibicka, K. P. (2017). Estradiol is a critical regulator of food-reward behavior. *Psychoneuroendocrinology, 78*, 193–202; Roney, J. R., & Simmons, Z. L. (2017). Ovarian hormone fluctuations predict within-cycle shifts in women's food intake. *Hormones and Behavior, 90*, 8–14.

28 **masculinized faces:** Roney, J. R., & Simmons, Z. L. (2008). Women's estradiol predicts preference for facial cues of men's testosterone. *Hormones and Behavior, 53*(1), 14–19.

28 **voices:** Pisanski, K., Hahn, A. C., Fisher, C. I., DeBruine, L. M., Feinberg, D. R., & Jones, B. C. (2014). Changes in salivary estradiol predict changes in women's preferences for vocal masculinity. *Hormones and Behavior, 66*(3), 493–97.

28 **behavioral displays:** Lukaszewski, A. W., & Roney, J. R. (2009). Estimated hormones predict women's mate preferences for dominant personality traits. *Personality and Individual Differences, 47*(3), 191–96.

28 **makes women look:** Tarumi, W., & Shinohara, K. (2020). Women's body odour during the ovulatory phase modulates testosterone and cortisol levels in men. *PloS one, 15*(3), e0230838; Schleifenbaum, L., Driebe, J. C., Gerlach, T. M.,

Penke, L., & Arslan, R. C. (2021). Women feel more attractive before ovulation: Evidence from a large-scale online diary study. *Evolutionary Human Sciences, 3,* e47.

28 *memory-forming version:* Leuner, B., & Shors, T. J. (2004). New spines, new memories. *Molecular Neurobiology, 29,* 117–30.

28 *neurotransmitters like serotonin:* Biegon, A., & McEwen, B. S. (1982). Modulation by estradiol of serotonin receptors in brain. *Journal of Neuroscience, 2,* 199–205; McEwen, B. S., Alves, S. E., Bulloch, K., & Weiland, N. G. (1997). Ovarian steroids and the brain: Implications for cognition and aging. *Neurology, 48*(5 Suppl 7), S8–S15.

30 *a mental health superhero:* Guennoun, R. (2020). Progesterone in the brain: Hormone, neurosteroid and neuroprotectant. *International Journal of Molecular Sciences, 21,* 5271.

30 *anti-inflammatory:* Chen, S., Wang, J. M., Irwin, R. W., Yao, J., Liu, L., & Brinton, R. D. (2011). Allopregnanolone promotes regeneration and reduces β-amyloid burden in a preclinical model of Alzheimer's disease. *PloS one, 6,* e24293.

30 *neuroprotective:* Gibson, C. L., Gray, L. J., Bath, P. M., & Murphy, S. P. (2008). Progesterone for the treatment of experimental brain injury: A systematic review. *Brain, 131,* 318–28.

30 *calm-inducing effects:* Brinton, R. D., Thompson, R. F., Foy, M. R., Baudry, M., Wang, J., Finch, C. E., Morgan, T. E., Pike, C. J., Mack, W. J., Stanczyk, F. Z., & Nilsen, J. (2008). Progesterone receptors: Form and function in brain. *Frontiers in Neuroendocrinology, 29,* 313–39.

30 *decreasing the risk of death by 50 percent:* Wright, D. W., Bauer, M. E., Hoffman, S. W., & Stein, D. G. (2001). Serum progesterone levels correlate with decreased cerebral edema after traumatic brain injury in male rats. *Journal of Neurotrauma, 18,* 901–909; Stein D. G. (2008). Progesterone exerts neuroprotective effects after brain injury. *Brain Research Reviews, 57,* 386–97.

30 *such as PTSD and alcohol use disorders:* Boero, G., Porcu, P., & Morrow, A. L. (2020). Pleiotropic actions of allopregnanolone underlie therapeutic benefits in stress-related disease. *Neurobiology of Stress, 12,* 100203.

31 *its calming metabolite ALLO:* Sundström-Poromaa, I., Comasco, E., Sumner, R., & Luders, E. (2020). Progesterone—Friend or foe? *Frontiers in Neuroendocrinology, 59,* 100856.

31 *neuroprotective effects:* Schumacher, M., Guennoun, R., Stein, D. G., & De Nicola, A. F. (2007). Progesterone: Therapeutic opportunities for neuroprotection and myelin repair. *Pharmacology & Therapeutics, 116,* 77–106.

32 *major depressive disorder:* Kornstein, S. G., Harvey, A. T., Rush, A. J., Wisniewski, S. R., Trivedi, M. H., Svikis, D. S., McKenzie, N. D., Bryan, C.,

& Harley, R. (2005). Self-reported premenstrual exacerbation of depressive symptoms in patients seeking treatment for major depression. *Psychological Medicine, 35*, 683–92.

32 ***personality disorders:*** Peters, J. R., Owens, S. A., Schmalenberger, K. M., & Eisenlohr-Moul, T. A. (2020). Differential effects of the menstrual cycle on reactive and proactive aggression in borderline personality disorder. *Aggressive Behavior, 46*, 151–61.

33 ***the functional connectivity:*** Arélin, K., Mueller, K., Barth, C., Rekkas, P. V., Kratzsch, J., Burmann, I., Villringer, A., & Sacher, J. (2015). Progesterone mediates brain functional connectivity changes during the menstrual cycle—a pilot resting state MRI study. *Frontiers in Neuroscience, 9*, 44.

37 ***see figure on previous page:*** Prior, J. C. (2020a). Women's reproductive system as balanced estradiol and progesterone actions—A revolutionary, paradigm-shifting concept in women's health. *Drug Discovery Today: Disease Models, 32*, 31–40.

Chapter 4: The Dawn of Bikini Science

40 ***relationship status:*** Rosenbaum, S., Gettler, L. T., McDade, T. W., Bechayda, S. S., & Kuzawa, C. W. (2018). Does a man's testosterone "rebound" as dependent children grow up, or when pairbonds end? A test in Cebu, Philippines. *American Journal of Human Biology, 30*(6).

40 ***having children:*** Gettler, L. T., McDade, T. W., Feranil, A. B., & Kuzawa, C. W. (2011). Longitudinal evidence that fatherhood decreases testosterone in human males. *Proceedings of the National Academy of Sciences, 108*(39), 16194–99.

40 ***a favorite sports team:*** Bernhardt, P. C., Dabbs, J. M., Jr., Fielden, J. A., & Lutter, C. D. (1998). Testosterone changes during vicarious experiences of winning and losing among fans at sporting events. *Physiology & Behavior, 65*, 59–62.

40 ***a favorite political candidate:*** Stanton, S. J., Beehner, J. C., Saini, E. K., Kuhn, C. M., & Labar, K. S. (2009). Dominance, politics, and physiology: Voters' testosterone changes on the night of the 2008 United States presidential election. *PloS one, 4*(10), e7543.

40 ***anticipating sex:*** Hamilton, L. D., & Meston, C. M. (2010). The effects of partner togetherness on salivary testosterone in women in long distance relationships. *Hormones and Behavior, 57*, 198–202.

40 ***a beautiful woman:*** Ronay, R., & Hippel, W. von. (2010). The presence of an attractive woman elevates testosterone and physical risk taking in young men. *Social Psychological and Personality Science, 1*, 57–64.

40 ***the presence of weapons:*** Klinesmith, J., Kasser, T., & McAndrew, F. T. (2006).

Guns, testosterone, and aggression: An experimental test of a mediational hypothesis. *Psychological Science, 17,* 568–71.

41 **research conducted on males:** Clayton, J. A., & Collins, F. S. (2014). Policy: NIH to balance sex in cell and animal studies. *Nature, 509,* 282–83.

42 **Our immune systems differ:** Breach, M. R., & Lenz, K. M. (2023). Sex differences in neurodevelopmental disorders: A key role for the immune system. *Current Topics in Behavioral Neurosciences, 62,* 165–206.

42 **regulate pain perception:** Galea, L. A. M., Choleris, E., Albert, A. Y. K., McCarthy, M. M., & Sohrabji, F. (2020). The promises and pitfalls of sex difference research. *Frontiers in Neuroendocrinology, 56,* 100817.

42 **Our brains differ:** Tabatadze, N., Huang, G., May, R. M., Jain, A., & Woolley, C. S. (2015). Sex differences in molecular signaling at inhibitory synapses in the hippocampus. *Journal of Neuroscience, 35,* 11252–65.

42 **estrogen-driven antibodies:** Zeng, Z., Surewaard, B. G., Wong, C. H., Guettler, C., Petri, B., Burkhard, R., Wyss, M., Le Moual, H., Devinney, R., Thompson, G. C., Blackwood, J., Joffe, A. R., McCoy, K. D., Jenne, C. N., & Kubes, P. (2018). Sex-hormone-driven innate antibodies protect females and infants against EPEC infection. *Nature Immunology, 19,* 1100–111.

42 **the cellular and molecular level:** Tabatadze, N., Huang, G., May, R. M., Jain, A., & Woolley, C. S. (2015). Sex differences in molecular signaling at inhibitory synapses in the hippocampus. *Journal of Neuroscience, 35,* 11252–65.

42 **fear of appearing sexist:** Clarke-Billings, L. (2016, November 29). Brain research hindered by scientists afraid of being called sexist, report says. *Newsweek.*

43 **drowsiness to cognitive impairment:** Zucker, I., & Prendergast, B. J. (2020). Sex differences in pharmacokinetics predict adverse drug reactions in women. *Biology of Sex Differences, 11,* 32.

43 **metabolize the drug much more slowly:** Greenblatt, D. J., Harmatz, J. S., Singh, N. N., Steinberg, F., Roth, T., Moline, M. L., Harris, S. C., & Kapil, R. P. (2014). Gender differences in pharmacokinetics and pharmacodynamics of zolpidem following sublingual administration. *Journal of Clinical Pharmacology, 54,* 282–90.

43 **forms of medical treatments:** Zucker, I., & Prendergast, B. J. (2020). Sex differences in pharmacokinetics predict adverse drug reactions in women. *Biology of Sex Differences, 11,* 32.

43 **new prescription drugs:** Simon, V. (2005). Wanted: Women in clinical trials. *Science, 308,* 1517.

43 **experience diagnostic delays:** Vlassoff, C. (2007). Gender differences in determinants and consequences of health and illness. *Journal of Health, Population and Nutrition, 25,* 47–61.

43 **automobile safety features:** Molinari, S., & Brooke, B. (2021, December 21).

Women are more likely to die or be injured in car crashes. There's a simple reason why. *Washington Post.*

44 **the "reasonable person" standard:** Buss, D. M. (2023). Sexual violence laws: Policy implications of psychological sex differences. *Evolution and Human Behavior, 44,* 278–283.

44 **research is not being done:** Galea, L. A. M., Choleris, E., Albert, A. Y. K., McCarthy, M. M., & Sohrabji, F. (2020). The promises and pitfalls of sex difference research. *Frontiers in Neuroendocrinology, 56,* 100817.

44 **only 5 percent of studies:** Rechlin, R. K., Splinter, T. F. L., Hodges, T. E., Albert, A. Y., & Galea, L. A. M. (2021). Harnessing the power of sex differences: What a difference ten years did not make. *bioRxiv,* 2021.06.30.450396.

47 **20 percent (!) of our cycle:** Stanhewicz, A. E., & Wong, B. J. (2020). Counterpoint: Investigators should not control for menstrual cycle phase when performing studies of vascular control that include women. *Journal of Applied Physiology, 129,* 1117–19.

Chapter 5: Understanding the Luteal Phase

55 **mood and stress regulation:** Turkmen, S., Backstrom, T., Wahlstrom, G., Andreen, L., & Johansson, I. M. (2011). Tolerance to allopregnanolone with focus on the GABA-A receptor. *British Journal of Pharmacology, 162*(2), 311–27.

56 **suppress our immune system:** Zwahlen, M., & Stute, P. (2024). Impact of progesterone on the immune system in women: A systematic literature review. *Archives of Gynecology and Obstetrics, 309,* 37–46.

56 **infection in the luteal phase:** Zwahlen, M., & Stute, P. (2024). Impact of progesterone on the immune system in women: A systematic literature review. *Archives of Gynecology and Obstetrics, 309*(1), 37–46.

56 **the end of the luteal phase:** Lee, H., Petrofsky, J., Shah, N., Awali, A., Shah, K., Alotaibi, M., & Yim, J. (2014). Higher sweating rate and skin blood flow during the luteal phase of the menstrual cycle. *Tohoku Journal of Experimental Medicine, 234,* 117–22.

56 **harder for bacteria and viruses:** Foxman, E. F., Storer, J. A., Vanaja, K., Levchenko, A., & Iwasaki, A. (2016). Two interferon-independent double-stranded RNA-induced host defense strategies suppress the common cold virus at warm temperature. *Proceedings of the National Academy of Sciences USA, 113*(30), 8496–501.

57 **7–11 percent more calories:** Zhang, S., Osumi, H., Uchizawa, A., Hamada, H., Park, I., Suzuki, Y., Tanaka, Y., Ishihara, A., Yajima, K., Seol, J., Satoh, M., Omi, N., & Tokuyama, K. (2020). Changes in sleeping energy metabolism and thermoregulation during menstrual cycle. *Physiological Reports, 8*(2), e14353.

57   *amino acids and lipids:* Draper, C. F., Duisters, K., Weger, B., Chakrabarti, A., Harms, A. C., Brennan, L., Hankemeier, T., Goulet, L., Konz, T., Martin, F. P., Moco, S., & van der Greef, J. (2018). Menstrual cycle rhythmicity: Metabolic patterns in healthy women. *Scientific Reports, 8*, 14568.

Chapter 6: Is There a Method to Your Madness?

64   *engaging with the outside world:* Laessle, R. G., Tuschl, R. J., Schweiger, U., & Pirke, K. M. (1990). Mood changes and physical complaints during the normal menstrual cycle in healthy young women. *Psychoneuroendocrinology, 15*, 131–38.

65   *Even female baboons:* Hausfater, G., & Skoblick, B. (1985). Perimenstrual behavior changes among female yellow baboons: Some similarities to premenstrual syndrome (PMS) in women. *American Journal of Primatology, 9*, 165–72.

67   **Meh, maybe next time:** Nesse R. M. (2000). Is depression an adaptation? *Archives of General Psychiatry, 57*, 14–20.

67   *feel unmotivated and blah:* Casto, K. V., Arthur, L. C., Lynch-Wells, S., & Blake, K. R. (2023). Women in their mid-follicular phase outcompete hormonal contraceptive users, an effect partially explained by relatively greater progesterone and cortisol reactivity to competition. *Psychoneuroendocrinology, 157*, 106367.

69   *protective against anxiety:* McHenry, J., Carrier, N., Hull, E., & Kabbaj, M. (2014). Sex differences in anxiety and depression: Role of testosterone. *Frontiers in Neuroendocrinology, 35*, 42–57.

70   *women in romantic relationships:* Reynolds, T. A., Makhanova, A., Marcinkowska, U. M., Jasienska, G., McNulty, J. K., Eckel, L. A., Nikonova, L., & Maner, J. K. (2018). Progesterone and women's anxiety across the menstrual cycle. *Hormones and Behavior, 102*, 34–40.

71   *the reactivity of the amygdala:* van Wingen, G. A., van Broekhoven, F., Verkes, R. J., Petersson, K. M., Bäckström, T., Buitelaar, J. K., & Fernández, G. (2008). Progesterone selectively increases amygdala reactivity in women. *Molecular Psychiatry, 13*, 325–33.

71   *increased vigilance to threat:* Pletzer, B., Crone, J. S., Kronbichler, M., & Kerschbaum, H. (2016). Menstrual cycle and hormonal contraceptive-dependent changes in intrinsic connectivity of resting-state brain networks correspond to behavioral changes due to hormonal status. *Brain Connectivity, 6*, 572–85.

71   *the number of connections:* van Wingen, G. A., van Broekhoven, F., Verkes, R. J., Petersson, K. M., Bäckström, T., Buitelaar, J. K., & Fernández, G. (2008). Progesterone selectively increases amygdala reactivity in women. *Molecular Psychiatry, 13*, 325–33.

71   *subtle signs of threat:* Maner, J. K., & Miller, S. L. (2014). Hormones and social

monitoring: Menstrual cycle shifts in progesterone underlie women's sensitivity to social information. *Evolution and Human Behavior, 35,* 9–16.
71 **possible sources of harm:** Wang, J., & Chen, A. (2020). High progesterone levels facilitate women's social information processing by optimizing attention allocation. *Psychoneuroendocrinology, 122,* 104882.
73 **cycle-related mood changes:** Haywood, A., Slade, P., & King, H. (2007). Psychosocial associates of premenstrual symptoms and the moderating role of social support in a community sample. *Journal of Psychosomatic Research, 62,* 9–13.
73 **pressure from work:** Kuczmierczyk, A. R., Labrum, A. H., & Johnson, C. C. (1992). Perception of family and work environments in women with premenstrual syndrome. *Journal of Psychosomatic Research, 36,* 787–95.
74 **women's work-based productivity:** Hardie, E. A. (1997). PMS in the workplace: Dispelling the myth of cyclic dysfunction. *Journal of Occupational and Organizational Psychology, 70,* 97–102.
74 **research suggests that we can feel:** Ussher, J. M., & Perz, J. (2013). PMS as a process of negotiation: Women's experience and management of premenstrual distress. *Psychology & Health, 28*(8), 909–27.
74 **chronic stress has created:** Granda, D., Szmidt, M. K., & Kaluza, J. (2021). Is premenstrual syndrome associated with inflammation, oxidative stress and antioxidant status? A systematic review of case-control and cross-sectional studies. *Antioxidants, 10,* 604.
75 **an emphasis on plants:** Katz, D. L., & Meller, S. (2014). Can we say what diet is best for health? *Annual Review of Public Health, 35,* 83–103.
75 **staying physically active:** Hötting, K., & Röder, B. (2013). Beneficial effects of physical exercise on neuroplasticity and cognition. *Neuroscience and Biobehavioral Reviews, 37,* 2243–57.
75 **managing our stress:** Pittenger, C., & Duman, R. S. (2008). Stress, depression, and neuroplasticity: A convergence of mechanisms. *Neuropsychopharmacology, 33,* 88–109.
75 **nurturing our relationships:** Serra, M., Pisu, M. G., Mostallino, M. C., Sanna, E., & Biggio, G. (2008). Changes in neuroactive steroid content during social isolation stress modulate GABAA receptor plasticity and function. *Brain Research Reviews, 57,* 520–30.
75 **getting enough sleep:** Stee, W., & Peigneux, P. (2021). Post-learning micro- and macro-structural neuroplasticity changes with time and sleep. *Biochemical Pharmacology, 191,* 114369.
75 **and sunlight:** Costello, A., Linning-Duffy, K., Vandenbrook, C., Lonstein, J. S., & Yan, L. (2023). Effects of bright light therapy on neuroinflammatory and neuroplasticity markers in a diurnal rodent model of seasonal affective disorder. *Annals of Medicine, 55,* 2249015.

76 *hormonal changes across the cycle:* Kiesner, J., & Pastore, M. (2010). Day-to-day co-variations of psychological and physical symptoms of the menstrual cycle: Insights to individual differences in steroid reactivity. *Psychoneuroendocrinology, 35,* 350–63.

78 *exercise is a huge game changer:* Prior, J. C., Vigna, Y., Sciarretta, D., Alojado, N., & Schulzer, M. (1987). Conditioning exercise decreases premenstrual symptoms: A prospective, controlled 6-month trial. *Fertility and Sterility, 47,* 402–8.

78 *as effective as antidepressants:* Recchia, F., Leung, C. K., Chin, E. C., Fong, D. Y., Montero, D., Cheng, C. P., Yau, S. Y., & Siu, P. M. (2022). Comparative effectiveness of exercise, antidepressants and their combination in treating non-severe depression: A systematic review and network meta-analysis of randomised controlled trials. *British Journal of Sports Medicine, 56,* 1375–80.

78 *increasing well-being:* Miller, K. K., Perlis, R. H., Papakostas, G. I., Mischoulon, D., Losifescu, D. V., Brick, D. J., & Fava, M. (2009). Low-dose transdermal testosterone augmentation therapy improves depression severity in women. *CNS Spectrums, 14*(12), 688–94.

79 *Chasteberry (***Vitex agnus-castus***):* Csupor, D., Lantos, T., Hegyi, P., Benkö, R., Viola, R., Gyöngyi, Z., Csécsei, P., Tóth, B., Vasas, A., Márta, K., Rostás, I., Szentesi, A., & Matuz, M. (2019). Vitex agnus-castus in premenstrual syndrome: A meta-analysis of double-blind randomised controlled trials. *Complementary Therapies in Medicine, 47,* 102190.

79 *more mixed research support:* Moslehi, M., Arab, A., Shadnoush, M., & Hajianfar, H. (2019). The association between serum magnesium and premenstrual syndrome: A systematic review and meta-analysis of observational studies. *Biological Trace Element Research, 192,* 145–52.

80 *magnesium glycinate and magnesium citrate:* U.S. Department of Health and Human Services. (n.d.). *Office of Dietary Supplements—Magnesium.* NIH Office of Dietary Supplements.

80 *solid research support:* Mohammadi, M. M., Dehghan Nayeri, N., Mashhadi, M., & Varaei, S. (2022). Effect of omega-3 fatty acids on premenstrual syndrome: A systematic review and meta-analysis. *Journal of Obstetrics and Gynaecology Research, 48,* 1293–305.

80 *A recent meta-analysis:* Mohammadi, M. M., Dehghan Nayeri, N., Mashhadi, M., & Varaei, S. (2022). Effect of omega-3 fatty acids on premenstrual syndrome: A systematic review and meta-analysis. *Journal of Obstetrics and Gynaecology Research, 48,* 1293–305.

81 *to have calcium deficiencies:* Bahrami, A., Bahrami-Taghanaki, H., Afkhamizadeh, M., Avan, A., Mazloum Khorasani, Z., Esmaeili, H., Amin, B., Jazebi, S., Kamali, D., Ferns, G. A., Sadeghnia, H. R., & Ghayour-Mobarhan, M. (2018).

Menstrual disorders and premenstrual symptoms in adolescents: Prevalence and relationship to serum calcium and vitamin D concentrations. *Journal of Obstetrics and Gynecology, 38,* 989–95.

81 *calcium can improve mood:* Arab, A., Rafie, N., Askari, G., & Taghiabadi, M. (2020). Beneficial role of calcium in premenstrual syndrome: A systematic review of current literature. *International Journal of Preventive Medicine, 11,* 156.

81 *nondairy sources of calcium:* Maruyama, K., Oshima, T., & Ohyama, K. (2010). Exposure to exogenous estrogen through intake of commercial milk produced from pregnant cows. *Pediatrics International, 52,* 33–38.

81 *Vitamin B_6:* Wyatt, K. M., Dimmock, P. W., Jones, P. W., & Shaughn O'Brien, P. M. (1999). Efficacy of vitamin B-6 in the treatment of premenstrual syndrome: Systematic review. *BMJ, 318,* 1375–81.

82 *women's luteal-phase experiences:* Ussher, J. M., & Perz, J. (2013). PMS as a process of negotiation: Women's experience and management of premenstrual distress. *Psychology & Health, 28,* 909–27.

82 *our emotional regulation strategies:* Ussher, J. M., & Perz, J. (2011). PMS as a gendered illness linked to the construction and relational experience of hetero-femininity. *Sex Roles, 68,* 132–50.

82 *mood-related changes feel worse:* Ussher, J. M., & Wilding, J. M. (1992). Interactions between stress and performance during the menstrual cycle in relation to the premenstrual syndrome. *Journal of Reproductive and Infant Psychology, 10,* 83–101.

Chapter 7: Sex and Attraction on Progesterone

85 *ninety-seven women:* Marcinkowska, U. M., Shirazi, T., Mijas, M., & Roney, J. R. (2023). Hormonal underpinnings of the variation in sexual desire, arousal and activity throughout the menstrual cycle—A multifaceted approach. *Journal of Sex Research, 60(9),* 1297–303.

86 *sexual desire, sexual pleasure:* Ingram, C. F., Payne, K. S., Messore, M., & Scovell, J. M. (2020). Testosterone therapy and other treatment modalities for female sexual dysfunction. *Current Opinion in Urology, 30(3),* 309–16.

87 *the research lab twice:* Maner, J. K., & Miller, S. L. (2014). Hormones and social monitoring: Menstrual cycle shifts in progesterone underlie women's sensitivity to social information. *Evolution and Human Behavior, 35,* 9–16.

87 *Consistent with other research:* Racine, S. E., Culbert, K. M., Keel, P. K., Sisk, C. L., Burt, S. A., & Klump, K. L. (2012). Differential associations between ovarian hormones and disordered eating symptoms across the menstrual cycle in women. *International Journal of Eating Disorders, 45,* 333–44.

89 *lasting relationship satisfaction:* McNulty, J. K., Wenner, C. A., & Fisher, T. D.

(2016). Longitudinal associations among relationship satisfaction, sexual satisfaction, and frequency of sex in early marriage. *Archives of Sexual Behavior, 45*, 85–97.

90 *In one study, researchers:* Meltzer, A. L., Makhanova, A., Hicks, L. L., French, J. E., McNulty, J. K., & Bradbury, T. N. (2017). Quantifying the sexual afterglow: The lingering benefits of sex and their implications for pair-bonded relationships. *Psychological Science, 28*, 587–98.

91 *more sexually motivated:* Roney, J. R., & Simmons, Z. L. (2013). Hormonal predictors of sexual motivation in natural menstrual cycles. *Hormones and Behavior, 63*, 636–45.

91 *research finds when women:* Gangestad, S. W., Dinh, T., Lesko, L., & Haselton, M. G. (2023). Understanding women's estrus and extended sexuality, in Buss, D. M., *Oxford Handbook of Human Mating*. Oxford University Press, 700–738.

91 *researchers followed fifty:* Grebe, N. M., Gangestad, S. W., Garver-Apgar, C. E., & Thornhill, R. (2013). Women's luteal-phase sexual proceptivity and the functions of extended sexuality. *Psychological Science, 24*(10), 2106–10.

93 *our brain finds it rewarding:* Meston, C. M., & Buss, D. M. (2013). *Why women have sex: Understanding sexual motivations from adventure to revenge (and everything in between)*. Henry Holt and Company.

93 *10–40 percent of women:* Dunn, K. M., Cherkas, L. F., & Spector, T. D. (2005). Genetic influences on variation in female orgasmic function: A twin study. *Biology Letters, 1*, 260–63.

94 *all about your partner:* Grebe, N. M., Emery Thompson, M., & Gangestad, S. W. (2016). Hormonal predictors of women's extra-pair vs. in-pair sexual attraction in natural cycles: Implications for extended sexuality. *Hormones and Behavior, 78*, 211–19.

95 *it is traded off:* Trumble, B. C., Blackwell, A. D., Stieglitz, J., Thompson, M. E., Suarez, I. M., Kaplan, H., & Gurven, M. (2016). Associations between male testosterone and immune function in a pathogenically stressed forager-horticultural population. *American Journal of Physical Anthropology, 161*, 494–505.

95 *And several lines of research:* Roney, J. R., Simmons, Z. L., & Gray, P. B. (2011). Changes in estradiol predict within-women shifts in attraction to facial cues of men's testosterone. *Psychoneuroendocrinology, 36*, 742–49; Gildersleeve, K., Haselton, M. G., & Fales, M. R. (2014). Do women's mate preferences change across the ovulatory cycle? A meta-analytic review. *Psychological Bulletin, 140*, 1205–59.

96 *researchers had women interact:* Cantú, S. M., Simpson, J. A., Griskevicius, V., Weisberg, Y. J., Durante, K. M., & Beal, D. J. (2014). Fertile and selectively flirty: Women's behavior toward men changes across the ovulatory cycle. *Psychological Science, 25*, 431–38.

97 *research finds that monetary rewards:* Ossewaarde, L., van Wingen, G. A., Kooij-

man, S. C., Bäckström, T., Fernández, G., & Hermans, E. J. (2011). Changes in functioning of mesolimbic incentive processing circuits during the premenstrual phase. *Social Cognitive and Affective Neuroscience, 6,* 612–20.

100 **physical fitness and health:** Jiannine L. M. (2018). An investigation of the relationship between physical fitness, self-concept, and sexual functioning. *Journal of Education and Health Promotion, 7,* 57.

100 **finds that low sexual desire:** Mark, K. P., & Lasslo, J. A. (2018). Maintaining sexual desire in long-term relationships: A systematic review and conceptual model. *Journal of Sex Research, 55,* 563–81.

101 **evidence that self-compassion:** Siegel, J. A., Huellemann, K. L., Hillier, C. C., & Campbell, L. (2020). The protective role of self-compassion for women's positive body image: An open replication and extension. *Body Image, 32,* 136–44.

102 **Maca root:** Shin, B. C., Lee, M. S., Yang, E. J., Lim, H. S., & Ernst, E. (2010). Maca (L. meyenii) for improving sexual function: A systematic review. *BMC, 10,* 44.

103 **Tribulus terrestris:** Ghanbari, A., Akhshi, N., Nedaei, S. E., Mollica, A., Aneva, I. Y., Qi, Y., Liao, P., Darakhshan, S., Farzaei, M. H., Xiao, J., & Echeverría, J. (2021). Tribulus terrestris and female reproductive system health: A comprehensive review. *Phytomedicine, 84,* 153462.

104 **sexual desire dysfunction:** Canat, M., Canat, L., Öztürk, F. Y., Eroğlu, H., Atalay, H. A., & Altuntaş, Y. (2016). Vitamin D_3 deficiency is associated with female sexual dysfunction in premenopausal women. *International Urology and Nephrology, 48,* 1789–95.

104 **supplementing with vitamin D:** Krysiak, R., Szwajkosz, A., Marek, B., & Okopień, B. (2018). The effect of vitamin D supplementation on sexual functioning and depressive symptoms in young women with low vitamin D status. *Endokrynologia Polska, 69,* 168–74.

Chapter 8: Nutrition, Exercise, Sleep, and Recovery

106 **between 69 and 84 percent:** Runfola, C. D., Von Holle, A., Trace, S. E., Brownley, K. A., Hofmeier, S. M., Gagne, D. A., & Bulik, C. M. (2013). Body dissatisfaction in women across the lifespan: Results of the UNC-SELF and Gender and Body Image (GABI) studies. *European Eating Disorders Review, 21,* 52–59.

107 **neurons in our gut:** Kaelberer, M. M., Rupprecht, L. E., Liu, W. W., Weng, P., & Bohórquez, D. V. (2020). Neuropod cells: The emerging biology of gut-brain sensory transduction. *Annual Review of Neuroscience, 43,* 337–53.

109 **an extra 350–450 calories a day:** The caloric cost of pregnancy. (1973). *Nutrition Reviews, 31*(6), 177–79.

109 *an extra 500–700 calories a day:* Prentice, A. M., & Prentice, A. (1988a). Energy costs of lactation. *Annual Review of Nutrition, 8,* 63–79.

109 *naturally cycling women:* Zhang, S., Osumi, H., Uchizawa, A., Hamada, H., Park, I., Suzuki, Y., Tanaka, Y., Ishihara, A., Yajima, K., Seol, J., Satoh, M., Omi, N., & Tokuyama, K. (2020). Changes in sleeping energy metabolism and thermoregulation during menstrual cycle. *Physiological Reports, 8,* e14353.

111 *the average luteal-phase meal:* Gailliot, M. T., Hildebrandt, B., Eckel, L. A., & Baumeister, R. F. (2010). A theory of limited metabolic energy and premenstrual syndrome symptoms: Increased metabolic demands during the luteal phase divert metabolic resources from and impair self-control. *Review of General Psychology, 14,* 269–82.

112 *less sensitive to glucose:* Brown, S. A., Jiang, B., McElwee-Malloy, M., Wakeman, C., & Breton, M. D. (2015). Fluctuations of hyperglycemia and insulin sensitivity are linked to menstrual cycle phases in women with T1D. *Journal of Diabetes Science and Technology, 9,* 1192–99.

113 *finds that food craving:* Buffenstein, R., Poppitt, S. D., McDevitt, R. M., & Prentice, A. M. (1995). Food intake and the menstrual cycle: A retrospective analysis, with implications for appetite research. *Physiology and Behavior, 58,* 1067–77.

113 *binge eating:* Klump, K. L., Keel, P. K., Racine, S. E., Burt, S. A., Neale, M., Sisk, C. L., Boker, S., & Hu, J. Y. (2013). The interactive effects of estrogen and progesterone on changes in emotional eating across the menstrual cycle. *Journal of Abnormal Psychology, 122,* 131–37.

113 *disordered eating:* Gladis, M. M., & Walsh, B. T. (1987). Premenstrual exacerbation of binge eating in bulimia. *American Journal of Psychiatry, 144,* 1592–95.

113 *emotional eating:* Klump, K. L., Keel, P. K., Racine, S. E., Burt, S. A., Neale, M., Sisk, C. L., Boker, S., & Hu, J. Y. (2013). The interactive effects of estrogen and progesterone on changes in emotional eating across the menstrual cycle. *Journal of Abnormal Psychology, 122,* 131–37.

114 *single most powerful factor:* Bronson, F. H., & Manning, J. M. (1991). The energetic regulation of ovulation: A realistic role for body fat. *Biology of Reproduction, 44,* 945–50.

114 *polyunsaturated fatty acids:* Lassek, W., & Gaulin, S. (2008). Waist-hip ratio and cognitive ability: Is gluteofemoral fat a privileged store of neurodevelopmental resources? *Evolution and Human Behavior, 29,* 26–34.

114 *20 percent of the dry weight:* Del Prado, M., Villalpando, S., Lance, A., Alfonso, E., Demmelmair, H., & Koletzko, B. (2000). Contribution of dietary and newly formed arachidonic acid to milk secretion in women on low-fat diets. *Advances in Experimental Medicine and Biology, 478,* 407–8.

114 *isotope-labeled fatty acids:* Fidler, N., Sauerwald, T., Pohl, A., Demmelmair, H., & Koletzko, B. (2000). Docosahexaenoic acid transfer into human milk

after dietary supplementation: A randomized clinical trial. *Journal of Lipid Research, 41,* 1376–83.

115 ***a 66 percent decline in births:*** Stein, Z., Susser, M., Saenger, G., & Marolla, F. (1975). *Famine and human development: The Dutch hunger winter of 1944–1945.* Oxford University Press.

116 ***to put on lean muscle mass:*** Sung, E., Han, A., Hinrichs, T., Vorgerd, M., Manchado, C., & Platen, P. (2014). Effects of follicular versus luteal phase-based strength training in young women. *SpringerPlus, 3,* 668.

117 ***a 32 percent increase:*** Reis, E., Frick, U., & Schmidtbleicher, D. (1995). Frequency variations of strength training sessions triggered by the phases of the menstrual cycle. *International Journal of Sports Medicine, 16,* 545–50.

118 ***both humans and animal models:*** Sung, E., Han, A., Hinrichs, T., Vorgerd, M., Manchado, C., & Platen, P. (2014). Effects of follicular versus luteal phase-based strength training in young women. *SpringerPlus, 3,* 668.

118 ***Estrogen activates AMPK:*** Ikeda, K., Horie-Inoue, K., & Inoue, S. (2019). Functions of estrogen and estrogen receptor signaling on skeletal muscle. *Journal of Steroid Biochemistry and Molecular Biology, 191,* 105375.

118 ***inhibits protein breakdown:*** Oosthuyse, T., & Bosch, A. N. (2010). The effect of the menstrual cycle on exercise metabolism: Implications for exercise performance in eumenorrhoeic women. *Sports Medicine, 40,* 207–27.

118 ***boosts growth hormone:*** Jeukendrup, A., Saris, W. H., Brouns, F., & Kester, A. D. (1996). A new validated endurance performance test. *Medicine and Science in Sports and Exercise, 28,* 266–70.

118 ***takes a nose dive:*** Atukorala, K. R., Silva, W., Amarasiri, L., Fernando, D. M. S. (2022). Changes in serum testosterone during the menstrual cycle—An integrative systematic review of published literature. *GREM: Gynecological and Reproductive Endocrinology and Metabolism, 3,* 009–020.

119 ***metabolism, and respiratory drive:*** D'Eon, T. M., Sharoff, C., Chipkin, S. R., Grow, D., Ruby, B. C., & Braun, B. (2002). Regulation of exercise carbohydrate metabolism by estrogen and progesterone in women. *American Journal of Physiology. Endocrinology and Metabolism, 283*(5), E1046–55.

120 ***fifty minutes of endurance training:*** Pivarnik, J. M., Marichal, C. J., Spillman, T., & Morrow, J. R., Jr. (1992). Menstrual cycle phase affects temperature regulation during endurance exercise. *Journal of Applied Physiology, 72,* 543–48.

120 ***recent research reviews highlight:*** Pereira, H. M., Larson, R. D., & Bemben, D. A. (2020). Menstrual cycle effects on exercise-induced fatigability. *Frontiers in Physiology, 11,* 517.

Chapter 9: From PMS to Primary Care

128 *less tolerable in the luteal phase:* Riley, J. L., 3rd, Robinson, M. E., Wise, E. A., & Price, D. (1999). A meta-analytic review of pain perception across the menstrual cycle. *Pain, 81,* 225–35.

128 *neurotransmitters like GABA:* Smith S. S. (1994). Female sex steroid hormones: From receptors to networks to performance—Actions on the sensorimotor system. *Progress in Neurobiology, 44,* 55–86.

129 *nonprescription pain relievers:* Hart, K. E., & Hill, A. L. (1997). Generalized use of over-the-counter analgesics: Relationship to premenstrual symptoms. *Journal of Clinical Psychology, 53,* 197–200.

129 *like lupus and multiple sclerosis:* Sandyk, R. (1995). Premenstrual exacerbation of symptoms in multiple sclerosis is attenuated by treatment with weak electromagnetic fields. *International Journal of Neuroscience, 83,* 187–98.

129 *80 percent of lupus flare-ups:* Verthelyi, D. (2001). Sex hormones as immunomodulators in health and disease. *International Immunopharmacology, 1*(6), 983–93.

129 *women with rheumatoid arthritis:* Da Silva, J. A., & Spector, T. D. (1992). The role of pregnancy in the course and aetiology of rheumatoid arthritis. *Clinical Rheumatology, 11,* 189–94.

129 *fewer symptoms in the luteal phase:* Latman, N. S. (1983). Relation of menstrual cycle phase to symptoms of rheumatoid arthritis. *American Journal of Medicine, 74,* 957–60.

131 *premenstrual exacerbation (PME):* Pinkerton, J. V., Guico-Pabia, C. J., & Taylor, H. S. (2010). Menstrual cycle-related exacerbation of disease. *American Journal of Obstetrics & Gynecology, 202,* 221–31.

132 *Almost half of asthmatic women:* Tan, K. S. (2001). Premenstrual asthma: Epidemiology, pathogenesis and treatment. *Drugs, 61,* 2079–86.

132 *IBS, lupus, MS, and diabetes:* Goldner, W. S., Kraus, V. L., Sivitz, W. I., Hunter, S. K., & Dillon, J. S. (2004). Cyclic changes in glycemia assessed by continuous glucose monitoring system during multiple complete menstrual cycles in women with type 1 diabetes. *Diabetes Technology & Therapeutics, 6,* 473–80.

133 *obsessive-compulsive disorder:* Vulink, N. C., Denys, D., Bus, L., & Westenberg, H. G. (2006). Female hormones affect symptom severity in obsessive-compulsive disorder. *International Clinical Psychopharmacology, 21,* 171–75.

133 *eating disorders:* Nolan, L. N., & Hughes, L. (2022). Premenstrual exacerbation of mental health disorders: A systematic review of prospective studies. *Archives of Women's Mental Health, 25,* 831–52.

133 *almost 70 percent (!) of women:* Kornstein, S. G., Harvey, A. T., Rush, A. J., Wisniewski, S. R., Trivedi, M. H., Svikis, D. S., McKenzie, N. D., Bryan, C.,

& Harley, R. (2005). Self-reported premenstrual exacerbation of depressive symptoms in patients seeking treatment for major depression. *Psychological Medicine, 35*, 683–92.

133 **bipolar disorder:** Teatero, M. L., Mazmanian, D., & Sharma, V. (2014). Effects of the menstrual cycle on bipolar disorder. *Bipolar Disorders, 16*, 22–36.

133 **an average of 60 percent:** Price, W. A., Torem, M. S., & DiMarzio, L. R. (1987). Premenstrual exacerbation of bulimia. *Psychosomatics, 28*, 378–79.

136 **Researchers have also noted:** Yum, S. K., Yum, S. Y., & Kim, T. (2019). The problem of medicating women like the men: Conceptual discussion of menstrual cycle-dependent psychopharmacology. *Translational and Clinical Pharmacology, 27*, 127–33

136 **women's blood levels:** Carmassi, C., Del Grande, C., Masci, I., Caruso, D., Musetti, L., Fagiolini, A., & Dell'Osso, L. (2019). Lithium and valproate serum level fluctuations within the menstrual cycle: A systematic review. *International Clinical Psychopharmacology, 34*, 143–50.

136 **increasing lithium doses:** Conrad, C. D., & Hamilton, J. A. (1986). Recurrent premenstrual decline in serum lithium concentration: Clinical correlates and treatment implications. *Journal of the American Academy of Child Psychiatry, 25*, 852–53.

137 **suggested that women's anesthesia:** Nakagawa, M., Ooie, T., Takahashi, N., Taniguchi, Y., Anan, F., Yonemochi, H., & Saikawa, T. (2006). Influence of menstrual cycle on QT interval dynamics. *PACE, 29*, 607–13.

138 **finds that exposure therapy:** Pineles, S. L., Nillni, Y. I., King, M. W., Patton, S. C., Bauer, M. R., Mostoufi, S. M., Gerber, M. R., Hauger, R., Resick, P. A., Rasmusson, A. M., & Orr, S. P. (2016). Extinction retention and the menstrual cycle: Different associations for women with posttraumatic stress disorder. *Journal of Abnormal Psychology, 125*, 349–55.

140 **early stages of perimenopause:** Prior, J. C. (2018). Progesterone for treatment of symptomatic menopausal women. *Climacteric, 21*, 358–65.

140 **any cardiovascular risks:** Prior, J. C., Cameron, A., Fung, M., Hitchcock, C. L., Janssen, P., Lee, T., & Singer, J. (2023). Oral micronized progesterone for perimenopausal night sweats and hot flushes: A Phase III Canada-wide randomized placebo-controlled 4 month trial. *Scientific Reports, 13*, 9082.

141 **to be had from progesterone:** Prior, J. C. (2020). Women's reproductive system as balanced estradiol and progesterone actions—A revolutionary, paradigm-shifting concept in women's health. *Drug Discovery Today: Disease Models, 32*, 31–40.

141 **drug, alcohol, and nicotine cravings:** Fox, H. C., Sofuoglu, M., Morgan, P. T., Tuit, K. L., & Sinha, R. (2013). The effects of exogenous progesterone on drug craving and stress arousal in cocaine dependence: Impact of gender and

cue type. *Psychoneuroendocrinology, 38,* 1532–44; Lynch, W. J., & Sofuoglu, M. (2010). Role of progesterone in nicotine addiction: Evidence from initiation to relapse. *Experimental and Clinical Psychopharmacology, 18,* 451–61.

141 **estrogen does the opposite:** Moran-Santa Maria, M. M., Flanagan, J., & Brady, K. (2014). Ovarian hormones and drug abuse. *Current Psychiatry Reports, 16*(11), 511.

Chapter 10: When a Good Hormone Goes Bad

150 **startle more easily:** Bannbers, E., Kask, K., Wikström, J., Risbrough, V., & Poromaa, I. S. (2011). Patients with premenstrual dysphoric disorder have increased startle modulation during anticipation in the late luteal phase period in comparison to control subjects. *Psychoneuroendocrinology, 36,* 1184–92.

150 **called sensorimotor gating:** Kask, K., Gulinello, M., Bäckström, T., Geyer, M. A., & Sundström-Poromaa, I. (2008). Patients with premenstrual dysphoric disorder have increased startle response across both cycle phases and lower levels of prepulse inhibition during the late luteal phase of the menstrual cycle. *Neuropsychopharmacology, 33*(9), 2283–90.

150 **heightened negativity bias:** Rubinow, D. R., Smith, M. J., Schenkel, L. A., Schmidt, P. J., & Dancer, K. (2007). Facial emotion discrimination across the menstrual cycle in women with premenstrual dysphoric disorder (PMDD) and controls. *Journal of Affective Disorders, 104,* 37–44.

150 **regulate their emotional responses:** Petersen, N., London, E. D., Liang, L., Ghahremani, D. G., Gerards, R., Goldman, L., & Rapkin, A. J. (2016). Emotion regulation in women with premenstrual dysphoric disorder. *Archives of Women's Mental Health, 19,* 891–98.

150 **impairs women's cognitive control:** Comasco, E., & Sundström-Poromaa, I. (2015). Neuroimaging the menstrual cycle and premenstrual dysphoric disorder. *Current Psychiatry Reports, 17,* 77; Dubol, M., Epperson, C. N., Lanzenberger, R., Sundström-Poromaa, I., & Comasco, E. (2020). Neuroimaging premenstrual dysphoric disorder: A systematic and critical review. *Frontiers in Neuroendocrinology, 57,* 100838.

152 **the changes in GABAergic activity:** Hantsoo, L., & Epperson, C. N. (2020). Allopregnanolone in premenstrual dysphoric disorder (PMDD): Evidence for dysregulated sensitivity to GABA-A receptor modulating neuroactive steroids across the menstrual cycle. *Neurobiology of Stress, 12,* 100213.

152 **symptoms of withdrawal:** Hantsoo, L., & Epperson, C. N. (2015). Premenstrual dysphoric disorder: Epidemiology and treatment. *Current Psychiatry Reports, 17,* 87.

153 ***blunted serotonin production:*** Rasgon, N., Serra, M., Biggio, G., Pisu, M. G., Fairbanks, L., Tanavoli, S., & Rapkin, A. (2001). Neuroactive steroid-serotonergic interaction: Responses to an intravenous L-tryptophan challenge in women with premenstrual syndrome. *European Journal of Endocrinology, 145,* 25–33.

153 ***lower levels of serotonin circulating:*** Rapkin, A. J., Edelmuth, E., Chang, L. C., Reading, A. E., McGuire, M. T., & Su, T. P. (1987). Whole-blood serotonin in premenstrual syndrome. *Obstetrics and Gynecology, 70*(4), 533–37.

153 ***observed in healthy controls:*** Eriksson, O., Wall, A., Marteinsdottir, I., Agren, H., Hartvig, P., Blomqvist, G., Långström, B., & Naessén, T. (2006). Mood changes correlate to changes in brain serotonin precursor trapping in women with premenstrual dysphoria. *Psychiatry Research, 146,* 107–16.

155 ***nearly four thousand women:*** Pilver, C. E., Levy, B. R., Libby, D. J., & Desai, R. A. (2011). Posttraumatic stress disorder and trauma characteristics are correlates of premenstrual dysphoric disorder. *Archives of Women's Mental Health, 14,* 383–93.

155 ***6.7 times more likely:*** Perkonigg, A., Yonkers, K. A., Pfister, H., Lieb, R., & Wittchen, H. U. (2004). Risk factors for premenstrual dysphoric disorder in a community sample of young women: The role of traumatic events and posttraumatic stress disorder. *Journal of Clinical Psychiatry, 65,* 1314–22.

155 ***more than three thousand women:*** Bertone-Johnson, E. R., Whitcomb, B. W., Missmer, S. A., Manson, J. E., Hankinson, S. E., & Rich-Edwards, J. W. (2014). Early life emotional, physical, and sexual abuse and the development of premenstrual syndrome: A longitudinal study. *Journal of Women's Health, 23,* 729–39.

156 ***delayed cortisol awakening response:*** Hantsoo, L., Jagodnik, K. M., Novick, A. M., Baweja, R., di Scalea, T. L., Ozerdem, A., McGlade, E. C., Simeonova, D. I., Dekel, S., Kornfield, S. L., Nazareth, M., & Weiss, S. J. (2023). The role of the hypothalamic-pituitary-adrenal axis in depression across the female reproductive lifecycle: Current knowledge and future directions. *Frontiers in Endocrinology, 14,* 1295261.

156 ***a lower cortisol response:*** Hamidovic, A., Davis, J., & Soumare, F. (2024). Blunted cortisol response to acute psychosocial stress in women with premenstrual dysphoric disorder. *International Journal of Neuropsychopharmacology, 27*(3), pyae015.

156 ***in people with PTSD:*** Wessa, M., Rohleder, N., Kirschbaum, C., & Flor, H. (2006). Altered cortisol awakening response in posttraumatic stress disorder. *Psychoneuroendocrinology, 31,* 209–15.

156 ***and severe depression:*** Dedovic, K., & Ngiam, J. (2015). The cortisol awakening response and major depression: Examining the evidence. *Neuropsychiatric Disease and Treatment, 11,* 1181–89.

156 *problems with mental health:* Bannister, E. (2019). There is increasing evidence to suggest that brain inflammation could play a key role in the aetiology of psychiatric illness. Could inflammation be a cause of the premenstrual syndromes PMS and PMDD? *Post Reproductive Health, 25,* 157–61.

156 *elevated levels of inflammation:* Barone, J. C., Ho, A., Osborne, L. M., Eisenlohr-Moul, T. A., Morrow, A. L., Payne, J. L., Epperson, C. N., & Hantsoo, L. (2024). Luteal phase sertraline treatment of premenstrual dysphoric disorder (PMDD): Effects on markers of hypothalamic pituitary adrenal (HPA) axis activation and inflammation. *Psychoneuroendocrinology, 169,* 107145.

157 *American College of Obstetricians and Gynecologists:* Management of premenstrual syndrome: Green-top guideline no. 48. (2017). *BJOG: International Journal of Obstetrics and Gynaecology, 124,* e73–e105.

157 *symptoms of women taking SSRIs:* Freeman, E. W., Rickels, K., Arredondo, F., Kao, L. C., Pollack, S. E., & Sondheimer, S. J. (1999). Full- or half-cycle treatment of severe premenstrual syndrome with a serotonergic antidepressant. *Journal of Clinical Psychopharmacology, 19,* 3–8.

158 *nausea, insomnia, headaches:* Marjoribanks, J., Brown, J., O'Brien, P. M., & Wyatt, K. (2013). Selective serotonin reuptake inhibitors for premenstrual syndrome. *Cochrane Database of Systematic Reviews, 2013,* CD001396.

158 *when SSRI use is discontinued:* Csoka, A. B., Bahrick, A., & Mehtonen, O. P. (2008). Persistent sexual dysfunction after discontinuation of selective serotonin reuptake inhibitors. *Journal of Sexual Medicine, 5,* 227–33.

159 *citalopram:* Ravindran, L. N., Woods, S. A., Steiner, M., & Ravindran, A. V. (2007). Symptom-onset dosing with citalopram in the treatment of premenstrual dysphoric disorder (PMDD): A case series. *Archives of Women's Mental Health, 10,* 125–27.

159 *escitalopram:* Freeman, E. W., Sondheimer, S. J., Sammel, M. D., Ferdousi, T., & Lin, H. (2005). A preliminary study of luteal phase versus symptom-onset dosing with escitalopram for premenstrual dysphoric disorder. *Journal of Clinical Psychiatry, 66,* 769–73.

159 *fluoxetine:* Steinberg, E. M., Cardoso, G. M., Martinez, P. E., Rubinow, D. R., & Schmidt, P. J. (2012). Rapid response to fluoxetine in women with premenstrual dysphoric disorder. *Depression and Anxiety, 29,* 531–40.

159 *paroxetine:* Yonkers, K. A., Holthausen, G. A., Poschman, K., & Howell, H. B. (2006). Symptom-onset treatment for women with premenstrual dysphoric disorder. *Journal of Clinical Psychopharmacology, 26,* 198–202.

159 *sertraline:* Kornstein, S. G., Pearlstein, T. B., Fayyad, R., Farfel, G. M., & Gillespie, J. A. (2006). Low-dose sertraline in the treatment of moderate-to-severe premenstrual syndrome: Efficacy of 3 dosing strategies. *Journal of Clinical Psychiatry, 67*(10), 1624–32.

159 *mood and somatic symptoms:* Landén, M., Nissbrandt, H., Allgulander, C., Sörvik, K., Ysander, C., & Eriksson, E. (2007). Placebo-controlled trial comparing intermittent and continuous paroxetine in premenstrual dysphoric disorder. *Neuropsychopharmacology, 32*(1), 153–61.

159 *12 and 50 percent of women:* Halbreich U. (2008). Selective serotonin reuptake inhibitors and initial oral contraceptives for the treatment of PMDD: Effective but not enough. *CNS Spectrums, 13,* 566–72.

160 *drugs called SNRIs:* Ramos, M. G., Hara, C., & Rocha, F. L. (2009). Duloxetine treatment for women with premenstrual dysphoric disorder: A single-blind trial. *International Journal of Neuropsychopharmacology, 12,* 1081–88.

160 *Research finds that dutasteride:* Martinez, P. E., Rubinow, D. R., Nieman, L. K., Koziol, D. E., Morrow, A. L., Schiller, C. E., Cintron, D., Thompson, K. D., Khine, K. K., & Schmidt, P. J. (2016). 5α-reductase inhibition prevents the luteal phase increase in plasma allopregnanolone levels and mitigates symptoms in women with premenstrual dysphoric disorder. *Neuropsychopharmacology, 41,* 1093–102.

161 *progestin drospirenone (3 milligrams):* Marr, J., Heinemann, K., Kunz, M., & Rapkin, A. (2011). Ethinyl estradiol 20μg/drospirenone 3mg 24/4 oral contraceptive for the treatment of functional impairment in women with premenstrual dysphoric disorder. *International Journal of Gynaecology and Obstetrics, 113,* 103–7.

161 *dosing of hormonal contraceptives:* de Wit, A. E., de Vries, Y. A., de Boer, M. K., Scheper, C., Fokkema, A., Janssen, C. A. H., Giltay, E. J., & Schoevers, R. A. (2021). Efficacy of combined oral contraceptives for depressive symptoms and overall symptomatology in premenstrual syndrome: Pairwise and network meta-analysis of randomized trials. *American Journal of Obstetrics & Gynecology, 225,* 624–33.

162 *the symptoms of PMDD:* Rapkin, A. J., Korotkaya, Y., & Taylor, K. C. (2019). Contraception counseling for women with premenstrual dysphoric disorder (PMDD): Current perspectives. *Open Access Journal of Contraception, 10,* 27–39.

162 *blocking progesterone receptors:* Comasco, E., Kopp Kallner, H., Bixo, M., Hirschberg, A. L., Nyback, S., de Grauw, H., Epperson, C. N., & Sundström-Poromaa, I. (2021). Ulipristal acetate for treatment of premenstrual dysphoric disorder: A proof-of-concept randomized controlled trial. *American Journal of Psychiatry, 178,* 256–65.

163 *more conventional treatments:* Freeman, E. W., Sondheimer, S. J., & Rickels, K. (1997). Gonadotropin-releasing hormone agonist in the treatment of premenstrual symptoms with and without ongoing dysphoria: A controlled study. *Psychopharmacology Bulletin, 33,* 303–9.

166 *help alleviate women's PMDD:* Kancheva Landolt, N., & Ivanov, K. (2021).

Short report: Cognitive behavioral therapy—A primary mode for premenstrual syndrome management: Systematic literature review. *Psychology, Health & Medicine, 26,* 1282–93.

166 **undergo CBT treatments:** Lustyk, M. K., Gerrish, W. G., Shaver, S., & Keys, S. L. (2009). Cognitive-behavioral therapy for premenstrual syndrome and premenstrual dysphoric disorder: A systematic review. *Archives of Women's Mental Health, 12,* 85–96.

166 **find similarly positive effects:** Busse, J. W., Montori, V. M., Krasnik, C., Patelis-Siotis, I., & Guyatt, G. H. (2009). Psychological intervention for premenstrual syndrome: A meta-analysis of randomized controlled trials. *Psychotherapy and Psychosomatics, 78,* 6–15.

166 **in-person appointments:** Borji-Navan, S., Mohammad-Alizadeh-Charandabi, S., Esmaeilpour, K., Mirghafourvand, M., & Ahmadian-Khooinarood, A. (2022). Internet-based cognitive-behavioral therapy for premenstrual syndrome: A randomized controlled trial. *BMC Women's Health, 22,* 5.

167 **a list of treatments:** Table adapted from Carlini, S. V., Lanza di Scalea, T., McNally, S. T., Lester, J., & Deligiannidis, K. M. (2022). Management of premenstrual dysphoric disorder: A scoping review. *International Journal of Women's Health, 14,* 1783–801.

168 **swimming:** Maged, A. M., Abbassy, A. H., Sakr, H. R., Elsawah, H., Wagih, H., Ogila, A. I., & Kotb, A. (2024). Correction: Effect of swimming exercise on premenstrual syndrome. *Archives of Gynecology and Obstetrics, 309,* 2957.

168 **Pilates:** Çitil, E. T., & Kaya, N. (2021). Effect of Pilates exercises on premenstrual syndrome symptoms: A quasi-experimental study. *Complementary Therapies in Medicine, 57,* 102623.

168 **yoga:** Dani, V., Vaghela, N., Mishra, D., & Sheth, M. (2019). To compare the effects of aerobic exercise and yoga on premenstrual syndrome. *Journal of Education and Health Promotion, 8*(1), 199.

168 **walking or dancing:** Witkoś, J., & Hartman-Petrycka, M. (2021). The influence of running and dancing on the occurrence and progression of premenstrual disorders. *International Journal of Environmental Research and Public Health, 18*(15), 7946.

169 **women who don't exercise:** Pearce, E., Jolly, K., Jones, L. L., Matthewman, G., Zanganeh, M., & Daley, A. (2020). Exercise for premenstrual syndrome: A systematic review and meta-analysis of randomised controlled trials. *BJGP Open, 4,* bjgpopen20X101032.

170 **effective at treating depression:** Kucia, K., Merk, W., Zapalowicz, K., & Medrala, T. (2019). Vagus nerve stimulation for treatment resistant depression: Case series of six patients—Retrospective efficacy and safety observation after one year follow up. *Neuropsychiatric Disease and Treatment, 15,* 3247–54.

170 *endometriosis:* Hao, M., Liu, X., & Guo, S.-W. (2022). Activation of α7 nicotinic acetylcholine receptor retards the development of endometriosis. *Reproductive Biology and Endocrinology, 20*(1).

170 *source of progesterone production:* Reid, R. L. (2012). When should surgical treatment be considered for premenstrual dysphoric disorder? *Menopause International, 18,* 77–81.

Chapter 11: Reclaiming Your Luteal Phase

180 *evidence of ovulation suppression:* Prior, J. C., Naess, M., Langhammer, A., & Forsmo, S. (2015). Ovulation prevalence in women with spontaneous normal-length menstrual cycles—A population-based cohort from HUNT3, Norway. *PloS one, 10,* e0134473.

181 *at work, school, or home:* Boivin, J., Sanders, K., & Schmidt, L. (2006). Age and social position moderate the effect of stress on fertility. *Evolution and Human Behavior, 27*(5), 345–56.

181 *lack of social support:* Dinh, T., Gangestad, S. W., Thompson, M. E., Tomiyama, A. J., Fessler, D. M. T., Robertson, T. E., & Haselton, M. G. (2021). Endocrinological effects of social exclusion and inclusion: Experimental evidence for adaptive regulation of female fecundity. *Hormones and Behavior, 130,* 104934.

181 *illness, inflammation, or vaccines:* Edelman, A., Boniface, E. R., Benhar, E., Han, L., Matteson, K. A., Favaro, C., Pearson, J. T., & Darney, B. G. (2022). Association between menstrual cycle length and coronavirus disease 2019 (COVID-19) vaccination: A U.S. cohort. *Obstetrics and Gynecology, 139*(4), 481–89.

181 *stress caused by wintertime!:* Shanmugam, D., Espinosa, M., Gassen, J., van Lamsweerde, A., Pearson, J. T., Benhar, E., & Hill, S. (2023). A multi-site study of the relationship between photoperiod and ovulation rate using Natural Cycles data. *Scientific Reports, 13*(1), 8379.

181 *it will shut down ovulation:* Schetter, C. D. (2011). Psychological science on pregnancy: Stress processes, biopsychosocial models, and emerging research issues. *Annual Review of Psychology, 62,* 531–58.

183 *fewer PMS symptoms:* Farasati, N., Siassi, F., Koohdani, F., Qorbani, M., Abashzadeh, K., & Sotoudeh, G. (2015). Western dietary pattern is related to premenstrual syndrome: A case-control study. *British Journal of Nutrition, 114*(12), 2016–21.

184 *lower depression and anxiety:* Tarı Selçuk, K., Avcı, D., & Alp Yılmaz, F. (2014). The prevalence of premenstrual syndrome among nursing students and affecting factors. *Journal of Psychiatric Nursing, 5,* 98–103.

184 *there is no research consensus:* Katz, D. L., & Meller, S. (2014). Can we say what diet is best for health? *Annual Review of Public Health, 35,* 83–103.

185 *summarized by Michael Pollan:* Pollan, M. (2024, April 2). *Unhappy meals.* https://michaelpollan.com/articles-archive/unhappy-meals/.
186 *the biggest barrier:* Katz, D. L., & Meller, S. (2014). Can we say what diet is best for health? *Annual Review of Public Health, 35,* 83–103.
190 *fewer PMS symptoms:* Bertone-Johnson, E. R., Hankinson, S. E., Willett, W. C., Johnson, S. R., & Manson, J. E. (2010). Adiposity and the development of premenstrual syndrome. *Journal of Women's Health, 19,* 1955–62.
193 *as effective as antidepressants:* Recchia, F., Leung, C. K., Chin, E. C., Fong, D. Y., Montero, D., Cheng, C. P., Yau, S. Y., & Siu, P. M. (2022). Comparative effectiveness of exercise, antidepressants and their combination in treating non-severe depression: A systematic review and network meta-analysis of Randomised Controlled Trials. *British Journal of Sports Medicine, 56,* 1375–80.
193 *mood-ruining inflammation:* Ren, J., & Xiao, H. (2023). Exercise for mental well-being: Exploring neurobiological advances and intervention effects in depression. *Life, 13,* 1505.
193 *It increases neuroplasticity:* Swain, R. A., Berggren, K. L., Kerr, A. L., Patel, A., Peplinski, C., & Sikorski, A. M. (2012). On aerobic exercise and behavioral and neural plasticity. *Brain Sciences, 2,* 709–44.
193 *keeps our brain sharp:* de Sousa Fernandes, M. S., Ordônio, T. F., Santos, G. C. J., Santos, L. E. R., Calazans, C. T., Gomes, D. A., & Santos, T. M. (2020). Effects of physical exercise on neuroplasticity and brain function: A systematic review in human and animal studies. *Neural Plasticity, 2020,* 8856621.
193 *regular physical activity:* Sanchez, B. N., Kraemer, W. J., & Maresh, C. M. (2023a). Premenstrual syndrome and exercise: A narrative review. *Women, 3,* 348–64.
193 *more regular ovulation:* Xie, F., You, Y., Guan, C., Gu, Y., Yao, F., & Xu, J. (2022). Association between physical activity and infertility: A comprehensive systematic review and meta-analysis. *Journal of Translational Medicine, 20,* 237.
193 *can mess with ovulation:* Mussawar, M., Balsom, A. A., Totosy de Zepetnek, J. O., & Gordon, J. L. (2023). The effect of physical activity on fertility: A mini-review. *F&S Reports, 4,* 150–58.
194 *getting good sleep:* Meers, J. M., Bower, J. L., & Alfano, C. A. (2020). Poor sleep and emotion dysregulation mediate the association between depressive and premenstrual symptoms in young adult women. *Archives of Women's Mental Health, 23,* 351–59.
194 *helps promote fertility:* Akamatsu, S., Otsuki, J., Fujii, M., Enatsu, N., Tsuji, Y., Iwasaki, T., & Shiotani, M. (2017). The poor quality of women's sleep negatively influences fertilization rates in assisted reproductive technology. *Fertility and Sterility, 108*(3).
194 *improving cognitive control:* Vanderlind, W. M., Beevers, C. G., Sherman, S. M., Trujillo, L. T., McGeary, J. E., Matthews, M. D., Maddox, W. T., & Schnyer,

D. M. (2014). Sleep and sadness: Exploring the relation among sleep, cognitive control, and depressive symptoms in young adults. *Sleep Medicine, 15*, 144–49.

194 *raising the threshold:* Simon, E. B., Oren, N., Sharon, H., Kirschner, A., Goldway, N., Okon-Singer, H., Tauman, R., Deweese, M. M., Keil, A., & Hendler, T. (2015). Losing neutrality: The neural basis of impaired emotional control without sleep. *Journal of Neuroscience, 35*, 13194–205.

194 *increasing neuroplasticity:* Gorgoni, M., D'Atri, A., Lauri, G., Rossini, P. M., Ferlazzo, F., & De Gennaro, L. (2013). Is sleep essential for neural plasticity in humans, and how does it affect motor and cognitive recovery? *Neural Plasticity, 2013*, 103949; Pickersgill, J. W., Turco, C. V., Ramdeo, K., Rehsi, R. S., Foglia, S. D., & Nelson, A. J. (2022). The combined influences of exercise, diet and sleep on neuroplasticity. *Frontiers in Psychology, 13*.

194 *supporting regular ovulation:* Lateef, O. M., & Akintubosun, M. O. (2020). Sleep and reproductive health. *Journal of Circadian Rhythms, 18*, 1.

194 *more likely to experience:* Jehan, S., Auguste, E., Hussain, M., Pandi-Perumal, S. R., Brzezinski, A., Gupta, R., Attarian, H., Jean-Louis, G., & McFarlane, S. I. (2016). Sleep and premenstrual syndrome. *Journal of Sleep Medicine and Disorders, 3*, 1061.

194 *exposure to direct sunlight:* Fleury, N., Geldenhuys, S., & Gorman, S. (2016). Sun exposure and its effects on human health: Mechanisms through which sun exposure could reduce the risk of developing obesity and cardiometabolic dysfunction. *International Journal of Environmental Research and Public Health, 13*, 999.

195 *synthesize vitamin D:* Irani, M., & Merhi, Z. (2014). Role of vitamin D in ovarian physiology and its implication in reproduction: A systematic review. *Fertility and Sterility, 102*, 460–68.e3.

195 *suppress melatonin production:* Roenneberg, T., & Merrow, M. (2005). Circadian clocks—The fall and rise of physiology. *Nature Reviews. Molecular Cell Biology, 6*, 965–71.

195 *artificial light at inappropriate times:* Moralia, M. A., Quignon, C., Simonneaux, M., & Simonneaux, V. (2022). Environmental disruption of reproductive rhythms. *Frontiers in Neuroendocrinology, 66*, 100990.

195 *night-shift work was associated:* Lawson, C. C., Whelan, E. A., Lividoti Hibert, E. N., Spiegelman, D., Schernhammer, E. S., & Rich-Edwards, J. W. (2011). Rotating shift work and menstrual cycle characteristics. *Epidemiology, 22*(3), 305–12.

195 *recent systematic review:* Cai, C., Vandermeer, B., Khurana, R., Nerenberg, K., Featherstone, R., Sebastianski, M., & Davenport, M. H. (2019). The impact of occupational shift work and working hours during pregnancy on health out-

comes: A systematic review and meta-analysis. *American Journal of Obstetrics & Gynecology, 221*(6), 563–76.

196 *avoiding alcohol altogether:* Fernández, M. D. M., Saulyte, J., Inskip, H. M., & Takkouche, B. (2018). Premenstrual syndrome and alcohol consumption: A systematic review and meta-analysis. *BMJ Open, 8*(3), e019490.

196 *can disrupt ovulation:* Van Voorhis, B. J., Syrop, C. H., Hammitt, D. G., Dunn, M. S., & Snyder, G. D. (1992). Effects of smoking on ovulation induction for assisted reproductive techniques. *Fertility and Sterility, 58*(5), 981–85.

196 *if you are a smoker:* Choi, S. H., & Hamidovic, A. (2020). Association between smoking and premenstrual syndrome: A meta-analysis. *Frontiers in Psychiatry, 11*, 575526.

196 *researchers pooled data:* Fernández, M. D. M., Saulyte, J., Inskip, H. M., & Takkouche, B. (2018). Premenstrual syndrome and alcohol consumption: A systematic review and meta-analysis. *BMJ Open, 8*(3), e019490.

197 *heavy alcohol use:* Anwar, M. Y., Marcus, M., & Taylor, K. C. (2021). The association between alcohol intake and fecundability during menstrual cycle phases. *Human Reproduction, 36*(9), 2538–48.

197 *These results were echoed:* Fan, D., Liu, L., Xia, Q., Wang, W., Wu, S., Tian, G., Liu, Y., Ni, J., Wu, S., Guo, X., & Liu, Z. (2017). Female alcohol consumption and fecundability: A systematic review and dose-response meta-analysis. *Scientific Reports, 7*(1), 13815.

198 *having meaningful relationships:* Kiecolt-Glaser, J. K., Gouin, J. P., & Hantsoo, L. (2010). Close relationships, inflammation, and health. *Neuroscience and Biobehavioral Reviews, 35*(1), 33–38.

198 *supercharges the immune system:* Leschak, C. J., & Eisenberger, N. I. (2019). Two distinct immune pathways linking social relationships with health: Inflammatory and antiviral processes. *Psychosomatic Medicine, 81*(8), 711–19.

198 *healthy functioning of the HPA axis:* Hostinar, C. E., & Gunnar, M. R. (2013). Future directions in the study of social relationships as regulators of the HPA axis across development. *Journal of Clinical Child and Adolescent Psychology, 42*(4), 564–75.

198 *feel-good neurotransmitters:* Vitale, E. M., & Smith, A. S. (2022). Neurobiology of loneliness, isolation, and loss: Integrating human and animal perspectives. *Frontiers in Behavioral Neuroscience, 16*, 846315.

199 *less psychological turbulence:* Rezaee, H., Mahamed, F., & Amidi Mazaheri, M. (2015). Does spousal support can decrease women's premenstrual syndrome symptoms? *Global Journal of Health Science, 8*(5), 19–26.

199 *and less PMS:* Fontana, A. M., & Palfai, T. G. (1994). Psychosocial factors in premenstrual dysphoria: Stressors, appraisal, and coping processes. *Journal of Psychosomatic Research, 38*(6), 557–67.

199 **70 percent higher odds:** Schliep, K. C., Mumford, S. L., Vladutiu, C. J., Ahrens, K. A., Perkins, N. J., Sjaarda, L. A., Kissell, K. A., Prasad, A., Wactawski-Wende, J., & Schisterman, E. F. (2015). Perceived stress, reproductive hormones, and ovulatory function: A prospective cohort study. *Epidemiology, 26,* 177–84.

199 **(69.9 percent!!) had nonovulatory cycles:** Nagata, I., Kato, K., Seki, K., & Furuya, K. (1986). Ovulatory disturbances. Causative factors among Japanese student nurses in a dormitory. *Journal of Adolescent Health Care, 7,* 1–5.

199 **the SARS-CoV-2 (COVID-19) pandemic:** Barr, S., Bos, C., Goshtasebi, A., Kalidasan, D., Mercer, G. W., Shirin, S., & Prior, J. (2022). OR15-6 epidemic of subclinical ovulatory disturbances during SARS-CoV2 pandemic—An experiment of nature. *Journal of the Endocrine Society, 6*(Suppl 1), A682.

200 **stress in the follicular phase:** Dinh, T., Gangestad, S. W., Thompson, M. E., Tomiyama, A. J., Fessler, D. M. T., Robertson, T. E., & Haselton, M. G. (2021). Endocrinological effects of social exclusion and inclusion: Experimental evidence for adaptive regulation of female fecundity. *Hormones and Behavior, 130,* 104934.

200 **nearly 69 percent of women:** American Psychological Association. (2012, January 1). *2012 Stress by Gender.* https://www.apa.org/news/press/releases/stress/2012/gender.

200 **whether cognitive behavioral therapy:** Michopoulos, V., Mancini, F., Loucks, T. L., & Berga, S. L. (2013). Neuroendocrine recovery initiated by cognitive behavioral therapy in women with functional hypothalamic amenorrhea: A randomized, controlled trial. *Fertility and Sterility, 99,* 2084–91.e1.

201 **Mindfulness-based stress reduction:** Goldin, P. R., & Gross, J. J. (2010). Effects of mindfulness-based stress reduction (MBSR) on emotion regulation in social anxiety disorder. *Emotion, 10,* 83–91.

201 **stress, depression, and anxiety symptoms:** Chiesa, A., & Serretti, A. (2009). Mindfulness-based stress reduction for stress management in healthy people: A review and meta-analysis. *Journal of Alternative and Complementary Medicine, 15,* 593–600.

201 **Positive social connections:** Cohen, S., & Wills, T. A. (1985). Stress, social support, and the buffering hypothesis. *Psychological Bulletin, 98,* 310–57.

202 **expressive writing reduces stress:** Pennebaker, J. W. (1997). *Opening up: The healing power of expressing emotions* (rev. ed.). Guilford Press.

203 **we are well nourished:** Amon, M., Kek, T., & Klun, I. V. (2024). Endocrine disrupting chemicals and obesity prevention: Scoping review. *Journal of Health, Population and Nutrition, 43*(1).

204 **help your body clear EDCs:** Hong, L., Xu, Y., Wang, D., Zhang, Q., Li, X., Xie, C., Wu, J., Zhong, C., Fu, J., & Geng, S. (2023). Sulforaphane ameliorates bisphenol A-induced hepatic lipid accumulation by inhibiting endoplasmic reticulum stress. *Scientific Reports, 13,* 1147.

204 *ovulation actually occurred:* Malcolm, C. E., & Cumming, D. C. (2003). Does anovulation exist in eumenorrheic women? *Obstetrics and Gynecology, 102,* 317–18.

207 *high rate of false negatives:* Lynch, K. E., Mumford, S. L., Schliep, K. C., Whitcomb, B. W., Zarek, S. M., Pollack, A. Z., Bertone-Johnson, E. R., Danaher, M., Wactawski-Wende, J., Gaskins, A. J., & Schisterman, E. F. (2014). Assessment of anovulation in eumenorrheic women: Comparison of ovulation detection algorithms. *Fertility and Sterility, 102*(2), 511–18.e2.

208 *PdG levels above 5 µg/mL:* Wegrzynowicz, A. K., Beckley, A., Eyvazzadeh, A., Levy, G., Park, J., & Klein, J. (2022). Complete cycle mapping using a quantitative at-home hormone monitoring system in prediction of fertile days, confirmation of ovulation, and screening for ovulation issues preventing conception. *Medicina, 58,* 1853.

210 *new practices to become habits:* Gardner, B., Lally, P., & Wardle, J. (2012). Making health habitual: The psychology of 'habit-formation' and general practice. *British Journal of General Practice: Journal of the Royal College of General Practitioners, 62,* 664–66.

211 *called habit stacking:* Clear, J. (2018). *Atomic habits: An easy & proven way to build good habits & break bad ones.* Avery.

Chapter 12: The Future Is Sex Differentiated and Hormonal

218 *cause and prevent cancer:* Rubin, J. B., Lagas, J. S., Broestl, L., Sponagel, J., Rockwell, N., Rhee, G., Rosen, S. F., Chen, S., Klein, R. S., Imoukhuede, P., & Luo, J. (2020). Sex differences in cancer mechanisms. *Biology of Sex Differences, 11,* 17.

218 *respond to DNA damage:* Broestl, L., & Rubin, J. B. (2021). Sexual differentiation specifies cellular responses to DNA damage. *Endocrinology, 162,* bqab192.

218 *the molecular basis:* Lopes-Ramos, C. M., Chen, C. Y., Kuijjer, M. L., Paulson, J. N., Sonawane, A. R., Fagny, M., Platig, J., Glass, K., Quackenbush, J., & DeMeo, D. L. (2020). Sex differences in gene expression and regulatory networks across 29 human tissues. *Cell Reports, 31,* 107795.

224 **Dr. Claudia Barth:** Barth, C., & de Lange, A. G. (2020). Towards an understanding of women's brain aging: The immunology of pregnancy and menopause. *Frontiers in Neuroendocrinology, 58,* 100850.

224 **Dr. Emily Jacobs:** Martínez-García, M., Jacobs, E. G., de Lange, A. G., & Carmona, S. (2024). Advancing the neuroscience of human pregnancy. *Nature Neuroscience, 27,* 805–7.

224 **Dr. Lisa Mosconi:** Rahman, A., Schelbaum, E., Hoffman, K., Diaz, I., Hristov, H., Andrews, R., Jett, S., Jackson, H., Lee, A., Sarva, H., Pahlajani, S., Mat-

thews, D., Dyke, J., de Leon, M. J., Isaacson, R. .S., Brinton, R. D., & Mosconi, L. (2020). Sex-driven modifiers of Alzheimer's risk: A multi-modality brain imaging study. *Neurology, 95*:e166–78.

224 **Dr. Jerilynn Prior:** Prior, J. C. (2020a). Balanced actions of estradiol and progesterone—A new paradigm of women's reproductive health. *Drug Discovery Today: Disease Models, 32,* 27–29.

224 *changes in the brain:* Nehls, S., Losse, E., Enzensberger, C., Frodl, T., & Chechko, N. (2024). Time-sensitive changes in the maternal brain and their influence on mother-child attachment. *Translational Psychiatry, 14*(1).

226 **keep a mood diary:** Kiesner, J. (2011). One woman's low is another woman's high: Paradoxical effects of the menstrual cycle. *Psychoneuroendocrinology, 36,* 68–76.

227 **changes across the cycle:** Kiesner, J., & Pastore, M. (2010). Day-to-day covariations of psychological and physical symptoms of the menstrual cycle: Insights to individual differences in steroid reactivity. *Psychoneuroendocrinology, 35,* 350–63.

227 **each of us is a little different:** Lorenz, T. K., Gesselman, A. N., & Vitzthum, V. J. (2017). Variance in mood symptoms across menstrual cycles: Implications for premenstrual dysphoric disorder. *Women's Reproductive Health, 4,* 77–88.

227 **developing mood disorders:** Pereira, D., Pessoa, A. R., Madeira, N., Macedo, A., & Pereira, A. T. (2022). Association between premenstrual dysphoric disorder and perinatal depression: A systematic review. *Archives of Women's Mental Health, 25,* 61–70.

INDEX

abandonment fears, 59–61, 70, 72, 82–84
Ache population, 60–61
addictive behaviors
    processed foods and, 190
    progesterone and, 30, 141–42
    quitting in luteal phase, 144–45
adrenal gland, 155–56, 155n, 200
alcohol intake
    addiction to, 30, 141–42, 144–45
    during luteal phase, 125, 196–98
    sleep hygiene and, 194
allopregnanolone (ALLO)
    addictive behaviors and, 141–42
    biological reality of, 55
    mood changes and, 65, 74–75
    overview, 31–32, 152
    PMDD and, 151–53, 159, 160
    progestins and, 34–35, 142–43n
Alzheimer's disease, 139, 142–43, 217–18
Ambien (zolpidem), 43
amino acids, 57, 58, 124
amygdala, 28, 71, 83–84

animals
    hormone cycles, 65, 89–90
    PMS and, 7
    sex hormones, 15
antidepressants
    CBT comparison, 166
    cycle-dependent responses to, 136
    physical activity comparison, 78, 193
    for PMDD, 157–60, 173
    side effects, 103, 158, 158n, 193
anti-inflammatory foods, 179
anxiety
    animals and, 7
    defense system and, 76–77
    exercise for, 201
    during luteal phase, 92
    medication for, 160, 166
    mindfulness-based stress reduction for, 201
    nutritional support for, 184
    ovulation disturbances and, 199
    PMDD and, 150, 152
    progesterone and, 31–32, 34–35

anxiety (*cont.*)
   sex differences, 44
   testosterone and, 69
   threat sensitivity and, 68–72
   vagal nerve stimulation and, 170
asthma, 131–32
autoimmune diseases, 129, 140, 140n

baboons, 7, 65, 89
Barth, Claudia, 224
basal body temperature (BBT)
   cycle-phase dependent, 56–57, 56–57n, 110, 119–20
   exercise and overheating, 119–20, 125
   nighttime temperatures, 56–57n
   ovulation and, 204–5, 208, 211, 232
   pregnancy and, 56n, 57
   tracking tips, 232, 233
Beyond the Pill (Brighten), 239
bikini approach to research science, 38–50
   closing thoughts, 228–29
   cyclic effects absent from, 49–50, 135–39, 225–28
   end of, 216–24
   future and beyond, xiii–xiv, 224–25
   making females less female, 45–50
   maleness of being, 41–45
   overview, xi–xii, 38–41, 213–16
BIOptimizers, 236
bipolar disorder, 133, 133n
birth control pills. *See* hormonal birth control
bloating, 132–33, 160, 179

blood glucose fluctuations, 111–12, 112n, 124
blue-light-blocking glasses, 195
body fat, 69, 114, 203–4
body image issues, 106, 107
body temperature. *See* basal body temperature
bone health, 139, 163
brain effects
   book resources on, 239
   of estrogen, 16, 18, 25–26n, 26, 27–28, 142–43
   of female body fat, 114
   of menopause, 163
   overview, 10–12
   of progesterone, 22, 29–32, 55, 71, 139. *See also* mood changes
   of testosterone, 14
brain-ovarian axis, 181
breastfeeding, 109, 114
breast health, 141, 180
Briden, Lara, 19–20, 140, 238
Brighten, Jolene, 239
Brizendine, Louann, 238, 239

caffeine, 136, 144–45, 194
calcium, 81, 81n, 167
cardiovascular health, 139, 163
CBT (cognitive behavioral therapy), 165–67, 172, 200–201
cervix and cervical mucus, 26, 86, 205–8, 232
chamomile, 167, 179
chasteberry (*Vitex agnus-castus*), 79, 167
citalopram, 158n, 159
clinical outcomes studies. *See* bikini approach to research science

cognitive behavioral therapy (CBT), 165–67, 172, 200–201
communication with romantic partners, 82–84, 99–100
cookbooks and cooking websites, 187–88, 234–35
cortisol
   CBT's effect on, 200
   clinical outcomes studies on, 47–49
   PMDD and, 155–56
   stress response system and, 155n, 199–200
cramps, 178–79
cycle-based wellness. *See also* hormone cycle; resilience to hormonal change
   BIOptimizer supplements, 236
   book resources, 234–35, 238–39
   cycle-tracking guides and apps, 211, 225–28, 231–33, 237
   nontoxic workout wear, 237
   progesterone testing, 208–9, 237
cyclically changing health, 126–45
   chronic conditions, pain, and worsening symptoms, 128–35
   clinical outcomes and, 135–39
   overview, 126–28
   progesterone for health, 139–43
   things to do today, 143–45. *See also* cycle-based wellness; resilience to hormonal change

dairy products, 81n, 185
danger sensitivity, 68–72, 82–83, 130
defense (emotional change), 76–77
depression
   antidepressants drugs, 78, 103, 136, 157–60, 158n, 166, 173, 193
   birth control pills linked to, 34–35
   hallmark of, 67
   luteal phase symptom, 133, 133n
   progesterone and, 32
   testosterone and, 69
Donofrio, Jeanine, 234
dopamine, 11, 28, 66, 128, 141
drug metabolism, 43, 130, 135–37
dutasteride, 160, 160n
dysfunctional defense, 77
dysregulated defense, 76–77

eating disorders, 133, 133n
endocrine disrupters compounds (EDCs), 202–4, 237
endocrine system
   overview, 10–12, 11n
   sex hormones, 12–19. *See also* estrogen; progesterone; testosterone
endometriosis, 140, 161–62n, 170, 180
endurance training, 119–20, 121–22, 124–25
escitalopram, 158n, 159
estrogen
   addiction and, 141–42
   clinical research focus on, 142–43, 142–43n
   detoxification, 192
   follicular phase, 16–17, 18, 24, 40
   humorous description of, 140n
   muscle growth and, 118–22
   progesterone as counterbalance to, 140–41

estrogen (*cont.*)
  purpose of, xi, 15–16, 24–28, 25–26n
  sexual response and, 15–16, 15n, 24–28, 85, 94–96
estrogen-only cycle, 180–82
ethinyl estradiol, 161–62
Everyday Food (From the Kitchens of Martha Stewart Living), 235
evolution, 5, 5–6n, 13, 21, 22–23, 22n, 28, 30
evolutionary mismatch, 107–8
exercise and fitness
  cycle-based, 78, 116–25
  evolutionary mismatch and, 108
  for hormonal balance, 193–94, 209–10
  for period cramps, 179
  for PMDD symptoms, 168–69, 168n
  for stress management, 201
exposure therapy, 138
expressive writing, 201–2
extinction therapy, 214

fantasies, 101–2
feeling down (upside of), 64–67. *See also* mood changes
Female Brain (Brizendine), 239
female sex hormones. *See* estrogen; progesterone
female sexual response, 85–105
  for connection, 88–94
  estrogen and, 15–16, 15n, 24–28, 85, 94–96
  lust, 94–98
  orgasms, 93
  overview, 85–88
  progesterone and, 86–88, 91–94, 96–97, 101, 130
  support for, 99–105
  testosterone and, 86, 95, 96, 98
fertility. *See* ovulation and fertility
fibroids, 180
Fifth Vital Sign (Hendrickson-Jack), 238
fish oil, 80
fitness. *See* exercise and fitness
Fix Your Period (Jardim), 19–20, 238
flaxseeds, 80, 179, 191, 192
fluoxetine, 158n, 159
fluvoxamine, 158n
follicular phase
  cheat sheet, 18
  estrogen and, 16–17, 18, 24, 40
  overview, 16–17, 18
  research done during, 46–49
  seed cycling during, 191
  stress during, 200
food preparation, 186–87, 188–89. *See also* nutritional support

GABA receptors, 31, 55, 65, 111, 141, 151–52
gender inequality
  overview, 38–41
  in research studies, 41–45. *See also* bikini approach to research science
gene-focused sex, 94–98, 94n
genetic risk factors, for PMDD, 156–57
ginger tea, 179
Glucose Goddess, 112, 124
gluteofemoral fat, 114

gonadotropin-releasing hormone (GnRH), 162–63, 200
Gottfried, Sara, 238
gut (slow-moving), 133
gut nutrient-sensing neurons, 107–8, 107n

habit stacking, 211
Hastings, Savannah, 170
healthy eating. *See* nutritional support
Hendrickson-Jack, Lisa, 238
herbal teas, 179
high-frequency strength training, 116–19, 121–22, 124–25
Hill, Maisie, 238
hippocampus, 28
hormonal balance, 177–212
    alcohol and, 196–98
    book recommendations, 238–39
    endocrine disrupters exposure and, 202–4
    movement for, 193–94
    nutritional support for, 183–92
    overview, 177–78, 182–83
    ovulation suppression with imbalances, 180–82
    ovulation tracking for, 204–9, 205n, 211, 232
    sleep for, 194–95
    smoking and, 196
    stress management for, 198–202
    things to do today, 209–12
hormonal birth control
    book resources, 35, 239
    for endometriosis, 161–62n
    how it works, 25n, 161–62n
    for PMDD symptoms, 160–62
    "progesterone" in, 34–35, 140n
Hormone Balance Bible, The (Tassone), 238
Hormone Cure, The (Gottfried), 238
hormone cycle
    cheat sheet, 18
    irregular cycles, 19–20
    overview, 10–12, 11n
    personal choices and, 20–23
    sex hormones, 12–19. *See also* estrogen; progesterone; testosterone
Hormone Intelligence (Romm), 238
Hormone Repair Manual (Briden), 140, 238
Hormone Reset Diet, The (Gottfried), 238
hormones. *See* cortisol; dopamine; estrogen; gonadotropin-releasing hormone; melatonin; oxytocin; progesterone; serotonin; testosterone; vasopressin
hydration, 179
Hypericum perforatum, 167
hypothalamic amenorrhea, 200
hypothalamic-pituitary-adrenal (HPA) axis, 155–56, 155n, 198–99
hypothalamus, 11, 16, 28, 155–56, 155n
hysterectomy, 147, 170

IAPMD (International Association for Premenstrual Disorders), 149, 171–72, 171–72n
IBS (irritable bowel syndrome), 130

immune system
    during luteal phase, 55–56, 61
    progesterone's effect on, 16, 129, 138, 140
    sex differences, 54, 55–56
    sexual response and, 95
    stress management and effect on, 198
    testosterone and, 95
    vaccinations and, 138
imperfectionism and perfectionism, 73–74, 189
inflammation
    alcohol and, 196–98
    cramping and, 178–79
    infections and, 56
    PMDD and, 153, 156
    progesterone and, 35, 129, 140
    smoking and, 196
    support for, 164, 169–70, 179, 193
insulin sensitivity, 111–12, 124
International Association for Premenstrual Disorders (IAPMD), 149, 171–72, 171–72n
In the Flo (Vitti), 239
irregular cycles, 19–20
irritable bowel syndrome (IBS), 130

Jacobs, Emily, 224
Jardim, Nicole, 19–20, 238

Kami-shoyo-san, 167

levonorgestrel, 161–62
LH (luteinizing hormone) test, 207, 209

Liddon, Angela, 234
lipids, 57, 58
Love and Lemons (Donofrio), 234
Love Real Food (Taylor), 234
low-frequency strength training, 116–19, 121–22, 124–25
lupus, 129
luteal phase
    advice overview, 106–8
    biological realities of, 54–62
    cheat sheet for, 18
    exercise advice for, 116–22, 124–25. *See also* exercise and fitness
    experiences versus symptoms of, 32–36
    immune changes, 129. *See also* immune system; inflammation
    metabolic changes, 130. *See also* metabolism
    nutritional advice for, 109–16, 123–24. *See also* nutritional support
    overview, 8, 17–19, 53–54
    pain perception during, 128–29, 128–29n
    premenstrual exacerbation, 131–35, 131n, 149
    progesterone and, 17–19, 29–30, 32, 40, 53–62. *See also* progesterone
    reclaiming, 177–212. *See also* hormonal balance
    respiratory drive changes, 119n, 130, 131–32
    seed cycling during, 190–92

sexual response during, 85–105, 130. *See also* female sexual response
upside to feeling down, 63–84. *See also* mood changes
luteinizing hormone (LH) test, 207, 209

maca root, 102–3
magnesium, 79, 79–80n, 167, 179, 236
Magnesium Breakthrough, 236
male sex hormone, 14–15, 15n. *See also* testosterone
MATE the Label, 237
MBSR (mindfulness-based stress reduction), 201
medical conditions exacerbated by progesterone, 133, 133n, 143–44
medical research. *See* bikini approach to research science
melatonin, 194, 195, 236
menopause
  book resources, 238
  early menopause health risks, 170
  exercise advice for, 214n
  future research directions for, 224–25
  health effects of, 163
  hormone replacement therapy for, 140, 142–43n, 143
  PMDD symptom resolution at, 148
Menopause Brain, The (Mosconi), 238
menstrual cramps, 178–79
mental health symptoms, 30–32, 63–84, 133. *See also* mood changes

metabolism
  of alcohol, 197–98
  cycle differences, 33, 109–10
  of drugs, 43, 130, 135–37
  luteal phase changes, 57–59, 119, 130
  sex differences, 42, 43
micronized progesterone, 140n, 145, 145n
mindfulness-based stress reduction (MBSR), 201
minimalistbaker.com, 235
Mira Hormone Monitor, 208–9
mittelschmerz, 178–79
mood changes (luteal phase), 63–84
  dysregulation and dysfunction of defenses, 72–75
  overview, 63–64
  stress response system and, 154–57
  testosterone and, 69
  things to do today, 75–84
  threat sensitivity and, 68–72, 76, 130
  upside to feeling down, 64–67
mood tracking, 75–76
Mosconi, Lisa, 224, 238, 239
motherhood, 20–22. *See also* postpartum; pregnancy
motivational state, during luteal phase, 66–67, 66n, 72
movement. *See* exercise and fitness
multiple sclerosis (MS), 129, 129n
muscle growth, 116–22
myo-inositol, 167

Natural Cycles, 25–26
natural cycling, defined, 25n

natural selection, 5, 5–6n, 13, 21, 22, 22n
negativity bias, 150–51
nervous system, estrogen's effect on, 28, 128–29, 128–29n, 169–70
nondairy products, 81, 81n
"normal," 3, 45, 223
nutrient-sensing neurons (neuropods), 107–8, 107n
nutritional support
    cookbooks and cooking websites, 187–88, 234–35
    embracing imperfectionism, 189
    evolutionary mismatch and, 107–8
    food preparation, 186–87, 188–89
    go-to items, 189–90
    for hormonal balance, 183–92, 209–10
    leftovers, 188
    during luteal phase, 57–59, 59n, 109–16
    menus, 188
    overview, 183–86, 203–4
    for resilience to hormonal changes, 78–79
    seed cycling, 190–92
    for sexual function, 102–5
    tracking cycle with hunger and food intake, 122–24

obsessive compulsive disorder (OCD), 133, 133n
Oh She Glows Cookbook, The (Liddon), 234
omega-3 fatty acids, 80, 167, 179
oral contraceptives. *See* hormonal birth control
orgasms, 93
ovary removal, 170
ovulation and fertility
    follicular phase and, 16–17, 18
    identification of, 20
    nutritional support for, 113–14
    support for, 145, 182–204. *See also* resilience to hormonal change
    tracking, 204–9, 205n, 211, 232
ovulation suppression, 140n, 180–82, 199
oxytocin, 11, 90, 92

pain perception, 128–29, 128–29n
panic disorder, 133, 133n
paroxetine, 158n, 159
PCOS (polycystic ovarian syndrome), 19
peppermint tea, 179
perception, 68–72, 130
perfectionism, 73–74, 189
perimenopause
    book resources, 238
    exercise advice for, 214n
    future research directions for, 224–25
    irregular cycles and, 19
    PMDD and, 151n
    relief during, 20, 140
Perimenopause Power (Hill), 238
period cramps, 178–79
Period Power (Hill), 238
Period Repair Manual (Briden), 19–20, 238
PGR (progesterone receptor gene), 157
pituitary, 11, 16

Index

plant-based diet, 185, 204, 234
pleasure, 27–28, 65–67, 66n, 86, 97, 130, 190
PMDD. *See* premenstrual dysphoric disorder
PMDD cycle-tracking calendar, 171–72
PME (premenstrual exacerbation), 131–35, 131n, 149
PMS (premenstrual syndrome)
    experiences versus symptoms of, 32–36
    luteal phase and, 18
    overview, ix–xi, 3–9, 5–6n, 16
    PMDD comparison, 133n
    progesterone and, 29–30, 29n, 31
    rethinking, 8, 29–30, 29n, 36. *See also* mood changes
    treatment and support for, 167–68, 168n, 182–204. *See also* exercise and fitness; nutritional support
Pollan, Michael, 185
polycystic ovarian syndrome (PCOS), 19
postpartum, 151n, 224–25, 227
post-SSRI sexual dysfunction (PSSD), 158, 158n
posttraumatic stress disorder (PTSD), 30, 133, 133n, 138, 156
prairie voles, 89–90
prefrontal cortex, 28
pregnancy
    basal body temperature and, 56n
    biological realities of luteal phase for, 53–54, 56–62
    future research directions for, 224–25

    immune system changes and, 129
    luteal phase and, 17, 18, 19
    nutritional changes, 109, 113–15
    overview, 12, 15–19, 24–26, 25n, 28–30
    ovulation suppression and, 181, 199
    pain perception changes and, 128–29
    threat sensitivity and, 70, 71–72, 76, 130
premenstrual dysphoric disorder (PMDD), 146–74
    causes of, 150–57
    differential diagnosis, 149
    drug-free treatments, 163–70
    medications for, 157–63, 173–74
    overview, 77, 134, 146–50
    PME comparison, 133n
    suicide risk and, 6
    symptoms and diagnostic criteria, 148–49, 171
    things to do today, 170–74
premenstrual exacerbation (PME), 131–35, 131n, 149
premenstrual syndrome. *See* PMS
Prior, Jerilynn, 224, 231
processed foods, 114–15, 183–84, 185, 190
progesterone
    addiction and, 141–42
    estrogen as counterbalance to, 140–41
    "in" hormonal birth control, 34–35, 140n
    immune system and, 16, 129, 138, 140

progesterone (*cont.*)
    luteal phase, 17–19, 29–30, 32, 40, 53–62. *See also* luteal phase
    micronized progesterone, 140n, 145, 145n
    muscle growth and, 118–22
    pain perception and, 128–29, 128n
    PMDD and, 151, 151n
    PMS and, 8, 29–30, 29n, 36. *See also* mood changes
    positive health effects of, 139–43
    purpose of, xi, 16, 24, 29–31
    smooth muscle relaxation, 129–30
    testing levels of, 208–9, 237
progesterone-blocking treatments, 162–63
progesterone receptor gene (PGR), 157
progestin drospirenone, 161
progestins, 34–35, 142–43n, 160–62
Proov (progesterone test), 208–9, 237
protein intake, 123–24, 185
Prozac, 157–58
PSSD (post-SSRI sexual dysfunction), 158, 158n
PTSD (posttraumatic stress disorder), 30, 133, 133n, 138, 156
pumpkin seeds, 191, 192

recommendations
    cookbooks and cooking websites, 234–35
    for cycle tracking, 231–33
    hormone books, 238–39
    supplements, 236–37
    wellness app, 237
relationship health and communication, 82–84, 99–101
research. *See* bikini approach to research science
resilience to hormonal change, 182–204
    endocrine disrupters exposure limitation, 202–4
    movement for resilience, 193–94
    nutritional support, 183–92
    overview, 182–83, 209–12
    ovulation tracking, 204–9, 205n, 211, 232
    quitting smoking and reconsidering alcohol, 196–98
    sleep for, 194–95
    stress management, 198–202
resiliency practices, 75–84
resistance training, 69
respiration, 119n, 130, 131–32
rewards
    addictive behaviors and, 141–42, 196
    estrogen and, 27
    in luteal phase, 107–8
    pleasure versus rewards, 66n
    progesterone and, 66–67, 66n, 97, 196
Romm, Aviva, 238

saffron, 167
schizophrenia, 133, 133n
science. *See* bikini approach to research science
seed cycling, 190–92

selective serotonin reuptake
    inhibitors (SSRIs), 103,
    157–60, 158n, 166
self-care, 164–65, 173
self-kindness, 82
sensorimotor gating, 150
serotonin, 28, 66, 128, 141, 152–53,
    156–57. *See also* selective
    serotonin reuptake inhibitors
serotonin-norepinephrine reuptake
    inhibitors (SNRIs), 160
sertraline, 158n, 159
sesame seeds, 191–92
sex differences. *See* bikini approach to
    research science
sex hormones. *See also* estrogen;
    progesterone; testosterone
    overview, 12–13, 39–40
    purpose of, 13–16, 15n, 39
sexual response. *See* female sexual
    response
skin health, 139
SLC6A4 gene, 156–57
sleep, 66n, 69, 194–95, 209–10, 236
Sleep Breakthrough, 236
smoking, 144–45, 196
smooth muscle relaxation, 129–30
SNRIs (serotonin-norepinephrine
    reuptake inhibitors), 160
social abandonment fears, 59–61, 70,
    72, 82–84, 100
SSRIs (selective serotonin reuptake
    inhibitors), 103, 157–60, 158n,
    166
strength training, 116–19, 121–22,
    124–25
stress management, 145, 198–202,
    209–10

stress regulation
    cortisol levels and, 47–50
    metabolic resource availability
        and, 59
    overview, 12, 30–32, 55
    for ovulation support, 145
    perfectionism and, 73–75
    in PMDD, 154–57
    support for, 77–78, 145, 164–65,
        169, 198–202, 209–10
stress response system, 35, 154–57,
    169, 181
substance P, 128–29
suicide risk, 173–74
sunflower seeds, 191–92
sunlight exposure, 104, 164, 164n,
    194–95
supplements and vitamins
    for period cramps, 179
    PMDD treatment, 167–68, 169
    for resilience to hormonal
        changes, 78–82, 236–37
    for sexual function, 102–05
synthetic progesterone, 34–35,
    142–43n, 160–62

Tassone, Shawn, 238
Taylor, Kathryne, 234
testosterone
    fluctuation of, 40
    gene-focused sex, 95
    melatonin and, 236
    mood changes and, 69, 78
    purpose of, 14–15, 15n
theophylline, 136
This Is Your Brain on Birth Control
    (Hill), 35, 239
threat sensitivity, 68–72, 76, 130

TMJ, 144
trauma history, 155–56
traumatic brain injury, 30, 139
Tribulus terrestris, 103–4, 103n
28 Wellness app, 233, 235, 237

Upgrade, The (Brizendine), 238
upside to feeling down, 63–67. *See also* mood changes

vaccines, 138, 181, 181n
vagus nerve stimulation (VNS), 169–70
vasopressin, 90, 92
vitamin B_1, 167
vitamin B_6, 81–82, 167
vitamin D, 104–5, 167
Vitex agnus-castus (chasteberry), 79, 167

Vitti, Alisa, 239
VNS (vagus nerve stimulation), 169–70
voles, 89–90
vulnerable state, 68–72, 76, 130

water intake, 179
water retention, 133
wearable tech, 233
wellness app, 233, 235, 237
Woman Code (Vitti), 239
writing, 201–2

XX Brain, The (Mosconi), 239

zimelidine, 158n
zinc, 167
zolpidem (Ambien), 43

ABOUT THE AUTHOR

Sarah E. Hill, PhD, is the author of *This Is Your Brain on Birth Control* and an award-winning researcher who has spent most of her twenty-plus-year career studying women, relationships, and health. In addition to having established an award-winning health and relationships lab at Texas Christian University, she has published nearly one hundred academic research articles, is a sought-after public speaker, and sits on the scientific advisory boards for women's health companies such as Flo and 28 Wellness. Her research is regularly covered by national media, such as *The Washington Post*, *The New York Times*, and many others, and is regularly published in highly prestigious journals, including the *Journal of Personality and Social Psychology*, *Psychoneuroendocrinology*, *Psychological Science*, and *Health Psychology*.